The Hevert Collection

ORIGINS
of NATUROPATHIC
MEDICINE

In Their Own Words

GW00683552

The Hevert Collection

ORIGINS
of NATUROPATHIC
MEDICINE

In Their Own Words

Edited by SUSSANNA CZERANKO, ND, BBE

Foreword by RICK SEVERSON, PHD, MLS

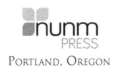

PORTLAND, OREGON

Original impression published by NCNM Press (2013)
ISBN: 978-0-9771435-2-8; 0-9771435-2-X

Front Cover Photographs
Center top: Benedict Lust, as a young man, overlaid on a photo of the
American Naturopathic School graduating class as it appears in the
October, 1906, issue of *The Naturopath and Herald of Health*.
Bottom cover photographs, left to right:
Henry Lindlahr, Ludwig Staden, Father Sebastian Kneipp,
Louis Kuhne, Adolf Just and Louisa Lust.

Back Cover Photograph
Lust Naturopathic Institute, p. 342.

NUNM Press
National University of Natural Medicine
049 SW Porter Street
Portland, Oregon 97201, USA
www.nunm.edu

Managing Editor: Nichole Wright
Production: Fourth Lloyd Productions, LLC.
Design: Richard Stodart

NUNM Press gratefully acknowledges the generous and prescient financial
support of HEVERT USA which has made possible the creation and
distribution of the *In Their Own Words* historical series.
The HEVERT COLLECTION comprises twelve historical compilations which
preserve for the healing professions significant and representational works
from contributors to the historical Benedict Lust journals.

Printed in the United States of America

ISBN: 978-1-945785-00-9
Library of Congress Control Number: 2016950600

Benedict Lust's courage and lifelong determination to build the
naturopathic profession and champion medical freedom are legend.
Seven decades after his death, he still inspires
Naturopathic doctors in many countries.

To him and to all those men and women, doctors, patients and
students alike who chose a different path to health,
this book series is dedicated.

TABLE OF CONTENTS

Dr. Sussanna Czeranko is passionate about naturopathy and its heritage in North America, so much so that she conceived this incredible project to reprise classic essays from Dr. Benedict Lust's early periodicals.

In 2010, Dr. Czeranko became the National College of Natural Medicine (NCNM) library's rare book room curator. Above all else, a curator is someone who cares for her charges (fragile books and journals in this case), like a physician would her patients. The rare book room—with its red oak cabinets, red walls, green door, patent medicine bottles and other worn down artifacts perched on shelves—has been resuscitated by its curator, and this series is the evidence.

Since this volume's essays pertain to naturopathy's history, it is fitting to begin with a few stories about the actual journals and place from which the readings have been painstakingly culled. From the point of view of NCNM's library, the story began in 1978. That is when Friedhelm Kirchfeld was hired as the first naturopathic medicine librarian in North America. Mr. Kirchfeld, a modest German immigrant who passed away in 2012, accepted the librarian position at NCNM while working in California for Cesar Chavez and the National Farm Workers Association. Wending his way to Oregon, Mr. Kirchfeld rescued hundreds of volumes of old homeopathy journals from the University of California San Francisco (UCSF) library. Those discarded volumes became the initial seed for NCNM's rare book room.

A co-author of *Nature Doctors* (NCNM Press, 1994, 2005), another historically important text for naturopathy, Mr. Kirchfeld worked tirelessly to gather an invaluable collection of books and journals from the old guard of retired and deceased naturopathic physicians. The crown jewel of that effort was receipt of the Benedict and John B. Lust collection from the John B. Lust estate in 1986.

The *Naturopath and Herald of Health* (formerly the *Kneipp Water Cure Monthly*) was published in New York by Benedict Lust from 1902–1915. The journal was published in separate German and

English editions from 1902-1907; both editions were combined in one volume beginning in 1908. The journal underwent another title change (actually just a title flip) in 1916—to the *Herald of Health and the Naturopath*—and ran under that title until 1957. It is from NCNM's rare book room copies of this journal, gifted from the Lust brothers, that Dr. Czeranko has recouped the essays gracing this series. Actually, that is not quite true.

In fact, the collection of *Naturopath and Herald of Health* issues (under its slightly varying titles) that came to NCNM from the Lusts had some missing parts, particularly for the years 1906 and 1907. Ever resourceful, Dr. Czeranko figured out that Bastyr University and Palmer College of Chiropractic had most of the missing issues, and she arranged for them to be scanned, bound, and added to the NCNM collection. A few of the essays in this series come from those originally missing issues.

It has been my honor to work with Dr. Czeranko these past few years. She is an excellent physician-scholar, steadfast in her passionate care and enthusiasm for naturopathy, its history, and its artifacts to be found in the NCNM rare book room. I thank Dr. Czeranko for undertaking this project, and I commend it to you as readers of these words from the past that are as relevant today as when they were first penned. You are welcome to visit our rare book room whenever you are in the Portland, Oregon area.

RICK SEVERSON, PhD, MLS
Library Director
National College of Natural Medicine
March 8, 2013

Preface

Researching an article drew me to NCNM's wonderful Friedhelm Kirchfeld Rare Book Collection, named in honor of NCNM's first, and late, beloved librarian, who understood how important it was and would be to protect these treasures. Various waves of donations which built the collection started when, acting on a tip, Friedhelm stopped in San Francisco on his way north to NCNM and was soon "dumpster diving" for discarded homeopathy volumes outside the library of the University of California [UCSF] in 1978. Contributions from individuals grew from there, such as the large donation from the estate of Dr. A.R. Hedges in 1982, and, powerfully, from the estate of Benedict Lust himself in 1985. Lust's library is the nucleus of the current collection. Over a thousand volumes contributed in the last two years alone from the Michael Chilton Library, for example, indicate the wishes of the profession and its friends to keep the literature vital for the community.

My first hour scouring delicately through that collection evolved into a determination to make the richness of these rare texts, histories, journals, magazines and artifacts available broadly to students and naturopathic doctors everywhere. My first stop that day was the "nature cure" shelves. There I rediscovered Benedict Lust and his many pioneering colleagues from a century ago. Three shelves display journals from 1896, the first year Benedict Lust began his publishing career, through 1945, the year he died. Within this historical naturopathic treasure trove are abundant, amazing topics, issues, ideas, historical details, testaments and predictions.

The articles reintroduced to our community in this collection come from that remarkable collection, arcing as it does back across a century and more. The *In Their Own Words* series is the tip of a fabulous, pristine iceberg of historical material, not floating around, but stopping in safe ports in docs' offices and students' desks more all the time. What is presented is actually a small selection of articles culled from Lust's journals, *The Kneipp Water Cure Monthly (1900-1901), The Naturopath and Herald of Health (1902-1915)* and *Herald of Health and Naturopath 1916-1923).*

Along the way, after reading more and more of the articles written more than 110 years ago, I was hooked. The pearls, insights and wisdom shone brilliantly on each page that I read. The experience was too good to hoard. I knew immediately that these books needed to be available for others, and soon. There is alarm in our profession about our roots and traditions bending and buckling in a world where allopathic medicine has most of the shelf space. We need to counter this dominance by making sure that the old literature is available and brings back into light these valuable insights into our roots: air, water, earth, sun and food.

This task of choosing the very best of the Naturopathic literature from over a century ago and of breathing new life into what our elders knew and shared widely with each other in those days was daunting. It takes persistence, lots of help and patience to convert intention on this scale into a beginning series reintroducing this magic knowledge into our complex, Standard of Care (SOC)-Primary Care Physician (PCP)-formulary-integrative medicine world. It has taken many like-minded people and their passion for a vision predicated on the 'Vis'. This first book in the *In Their Own Words* series is the result of a remarkable endeavor on the part of wonderful colleagues who felt as I do, that we must nurture our roots in this new, complex century to keep our philosophy and our mission alive, well and growing.

So many people have their fingerprints all over these pages. Without their hard work, this book would still be chugging along somewhere a thousand pages back. I am deeply grateful for the support of my colleague, Dr. Rick Severson, Friedhelm's successor and a fabulous librarian and archivist himself. His ears listened to my tales when I confronted obstacles along this journey. Dr. Severson would unclutter the path. To him, I am grateful for how he knows to convert a barrier into an opportunity, how to locate missing issues which were long felt to be lost (especially issues from 1906 and 1907). We got them, and thus the Benedict Lust journals collection at NCNM is now one specular, coherent and complete, unique collection. Rick never doubted this project for a nanosecond. His encouragement and guidance make him the rock star of naturopathic medical education library directors.

We have kept as closely as possible to the original text despite unusual but navigable grammar, punctuation and word use from that period. I want to acknowledge every NCNM student who typed or proof read articles while navigating their intense course loads and juggling their personal lives. Huge heaps of intense gratitude to *Allison Brumley, Angela Carlson, Avishan Saberian, Bonita Wilcox, Delia Sewell, Derek Andre, Derrick Schull, Joshua Corn, Katelyn Mudry, Katherine Venegas, Kimberly Kong, Kirsten Carle, Kyle Meyer, Lucy-Kate Reeve, Meagan Watts, Natalie Paravicini, Node Smith, Olif Wojciechowski, Rachel Caplan, Renae Rogers, Rhesa Napoli, Sarah Holloway, Tiffany Bloomingdale, Tina Dreisbach*, and all those whom I am inadvertently missing here. I so much enjoyed working with each and every student who sacrificed their scarce, precious leisure and play time for the hard work of meticulous research and transcription. As you launch yourselves into the Naturopathic profession, never forget how special and important your work has been. You have chosen a path of sacred work. I am especially indebted to the tireless work of **Dr. Karis Tressel** who was my diva of anti-chaos and who brought sublime organization and order to the colossal stacks of paper and minutia. Without Karis' exquisite, patient and detailed sense of clarity, I might still be searching in my stacks for that lost piece of paper.

I am very grateful for the unwavering, behind the scenes support of the Board of NCNM, Dr. Sandra Snyder, Susan Hunter, Nora Sande and Jerry Bores who have understood all along the importance of this project. I applaud Fourth Lloyd Productions, Nancy and Richard Stodart, my designers and coaches extraordinaire who guided me with alacrity every step of the way. Thank you!

Lastly, I want to thank my husband, David Schleich, who typically saw the ending from the beginning and much sooner than I could. He sees this first series as the first of a series of series. I think he may have a point because as you delve into this first book of twelve in series one, I am betting you'll be ready for more. May you enjoy these articles chosen from the past and from our elders *in their own words*.

Sussanna Czeranko, ND, BBE
Portland, Oregon. June 7, 2013

What is Naturopathy? will naturally be now asked by every one. Naturopathy embodies all natural healing methods, including Hydrotherapy (Priessnitz, Kneipp and Just's systems), Osteopathy, Heliotherapy (sun, light, and air cure), Hygienic and Physical and Mental Culture to the exclusion of all drugs and non-accidental surgery.

—Benedict Lust, *1902, 14*

Men and women who were guilty of no other offense than the giving of a bath or a massage, the instruction in dietetics or systems of exercise, were heavily and unmercifully fined or sent to jail.

—New York State Society of Naturopaths, *1914, 144*

The word "Naturopath" was the magic word that set us free. Although being a misnomer, it covered the subject. It has come to stay as a living protest against the autocracy, coercion, imposition, intolerance and persecution of the New York County Medical Society Trust in particular, and the American Medical Association Trust.

—Benedict Lust, *1921, 479*

INTRODUCTION

THE ORIGINS OF NATUROPATHIC MEDICINE

The story of naturopathic medicine is best told in the words of those who were there at the beginning; in the words, then, of those who established our profession. Our contemporary vantage point enables us to learn from those pioneers whose work constitutes our roots and traditions, if we know where to look. That same modern perspective can help us make changes and to sustain valuable modalities and ideas, particularly if we keep the history and original philosophy in mind. It is from those beginning years and from the surviving archives that we can learn much again, as if for the first time, about who we are.

Benedict Lust published abundantly and encouraged reflection, research and education among hundreds of colleagues. He was an editor of a number of Naturopathic journals, a valuable and important effort which spanned more than fifty years. His charisma, dedication and determination energized and guided other naturopaths to share in the creation of an emerging profession, a legacy which has persisted to the present. The contributions of Lust himself and of the early naturopaths can be found in the Benedict Lust Journals of that period: *The Kneipp Water Cure Monthly* (1900-1901); *The Naturopath and Herald of Health* (1902-1915); *Herald of Health and Naturopath* (1916 – 1957) and *Nature's Path* (1925-1960?).

Cumulatively and collectively, these serial publications contributed greatly to the formation of the naturopathic profession and became a voice for the many who increasingly joined its ranks. The first journal, *Amerikanischen Kneipp-Blätter* (1896-1899), edited by Lust, was written in German. In 1900 he launched an English edition, *The Kneipp Water Cure Monthly* , that was soon succeeded by a new health magazine, *The Naturopath and Herald of Health* which better addressed the interests of the growing number of Americans eager to learn more about naturopathic medicine. In January, 1902, a little over eleven decades ago, the first Naturopathic publication was literally hot off the press.

In many ways, the range of topics and issues debated and analyzed in these journals constitutes the history of the profession itself in these formative years.

The history of naturopathic medicine begins in 1896 in New York City four years after Lust's initial arrival in America. His first publication, *Amerikanischen Kneipp-Blätter*, as mentioned above, was in the German language. This publication advocated the wonders of Father Kneipp's water cure treatments. From these writings we know that the origins of naturopathic medicine precede the old world sanitariums of Vincent Priessnitz, Johann Schroth, Friedrich Eduard Bilz and Father Sebastian Kneipp. Numerous contributors in those early editions pointed back to Hippocrates, the father of medicine, and suggested that he was at the origin of an eventual naturopathic framework for medicine centuries earlier. Indeed, Priessnitz and others learned from Hippocrates and earlier healers that cold water was one of the best remedies for an array of presenting conditions. (Lust, 1900, 2) Although Hippocrates made bold statements about the importance of water, it was not until others, such as Paracelsus, that claims were published about the importance of nature in the healing process. Priessnitz (1799-1851), for example, studied nature and applied his observations clinically with great success. One of his remarkable contributions to medicine may well be his contention that "not the cold but the heat produced by cold water is the healing factor." (Lust, 1900, 2) Priessnitz, Schroth and Kneipp understood that tradition, and all healed themselves of debilitating injuries and disease with the use of cold water. Each of these men went on to establish large followings, sanitariums and the modest beginnings of what would soon become "naturopathic medicine" in North America, an *heterodox medical system* (Baer, 2002).

Benedict Lust, in addition to being a prolific editor and publisher, was also very catalytic on several fronts in the *professional formation* process. He was 20 years old when he first came to America and by age 24 had become an editor of his own health magazine. At 29 he founded the first U.S. Naturopathic College. The following year he created the first Naturopathic Association. He was fascinated with the "New World" and had come to America with ambitious ideas and ideals. At 22, despite living in the land of his dreams, the opportunities before him were eclipsed by a serious health condition; he was afflicted with deadly tuberculosis. He chose to return to Germany where he found Father Kneipp whose nature-cure interventions saved his life. Lust was profoundly affected by the miraculous recovery through Kneipp's water therapies and resolved to promote this life-healing, life-giving natural approach to primary care. He returned to America with many strategies and much energy to promote Father Kneipp's teaching and his work. (Lust, 1904, 145)

At the turn of the 20th century, there was a large German expatriate population in America, especially in the northeast. In those decades before WWI, these immigrants faithfully followed the customs of their mother country, such as the familiar and highly credible Kneipp "water cure". Even so, the Kneipp Cure was not broadly known or understood in America and some of its practices, such as barefoot walking, were met with skepticism at the very least, and sometimes with outright contempt and rejection. In fact, during this period of familiarization and the branding of "nature-cure", tensions inevitably arose among those who were advocating natural medicine. As in most processes of "professional formation", there emerged factions, based not only on philosophy, but also on tactics. In order to distance himself and his followers from one particular group, the somewhat fanatical 'Kneippianers', who had a much more confrontational and narrow strategy about building the profession, Lust formed the Naturopathic Society of America in New York City in September, 1902. (Lust, 1903, 37) The genesis of this organization was built on the intention of bringing together all the factions within a common framework to promote the broad goals of the emerging naturopathic wave.

In 1902, what we today know as "naturopathy" was not a coherent medical system. In fact, the very term, "naturopathy", was not understood nor systematized in terms of scope of practice, education or research support for its claims. This new word attempted to encompass "all natural healing methods, including Hydrotherapy (Priessnitz, Kneipp and Just's systems), Osteopathy, Heliotherapy (sun, light and air cure), Hygienic and Physical and Mental Culture to the exclusion of all drugs and non-accidental surgery." (Lust, 1902, 14) Lust described this framework with the term "naturopathy" and said of the label: "Naturopathy is a hybrid word. It is purposely so. No single tongue could distinguish a system whose origin, scope and purpose are universal—broad as the world, deep as love, high as heaven." (Lust, 1902, 32)

The word, 'naturopathy' was, as has been documented often elsewhere, coined by John H. Scheel who granted Lust permission to use it in conjunction with his new magazine. (Lust, 1902, 33) The mission of naturopathy at the outset was simple and powerful:

> We want every man, woman and child in this great land to know and embody and feel the truths of right living that mean conscious mastery. We plead for the renouncing of poisons from the coffee, white flour, glucose, lard, and like venom of the American table to patent medicines, tobacco, liquor and the other inevitable recourse of perverted appetite. (Lust, 1902, 32)

While the new naturopaths were committed to creating healthy people through life style reform, the gathering strength of the orthodox medical system, allopathic medicine, on the other hand, had a different agenda. Ostensibly, though, these biomedicine professionals had the wellbeing of the nation in mind. Claiming to want the best in public health, their approach was philosophically at odds with naturopathic medicine. The allopathic approach contemplated a system of treatment "which tries to effect by medicine the reversal of the symptoms characterizing a disease." (Bilz, 1900, 125) The opposition between the allopaths and naturopaths arose out of a differing understanding of "nature" and of the role of nature in human health and in the health of the planet. As Bilz explained at the turn of the century, the allopath "looks upon the symptoms of a disease as errors of nature, and endeavors to remove them by chemical means, not considering that in doing so the whole of the organic system gets disturbed and weakened in the [process]." (Bilz, 1900, 125) The emerging naturopathic profession, on the other hand, saw disease as a transgression of nature's laws. While the allopaths and their supporters could see looming large an unbelievably profitable pharmaceutical enterprise, the naturopaths were anchored in the roots and power of natural approaches to life-long wellness.

The differences among the allopaths and the naturopaths showed up most clearly in how each practiced his or her type of medicine. The naturopaths held strong convictions "that the laws of nature are necessary and eternal and that all phenomena in nature are but applications of immutable and universal principles." (Juettner, 1906, 225) Juettner argued that despite the curiosity "into the causes of the phenomena which the panorama of the living creation presents" (Juettner, 1906, 225) the practice of medicine did not live up to the ideals of inquiry and science. Medicine's dependence upon drugs was confounding for the Naturopaths. Juettner poses the following question, "Why the faith in the curative action of drugs taken internally should still survive among physicians is in itself a mystery as strange and singular as the lack of harmony among physicians concerning the use of drugs and the effects which are obtainable." (Juettner, 1906, 226) This enigma was especially perplexing when even medical doctors admitted "without hesitation that drug-medication is uncertain and disappointing." (Juettner, 1906, 227)

A compendium of citations and quotations by Medical Doctors assembled by Lust (Lust, 1906, p. 160) who shared the skepticism of the naturopaths on the merits of drugs, helped to corroborate and attach language to the growing reliance on toxic pharmaceuticals. In some ways, using the words of these MDs reinforced the naturopathic position on the evils of drug therapy. Examples of what these same MDs stated, "In many cases treated by physicians, chronic diseases have been subsequently brought about by the treatment of physicians." (Dieser, 1906, 160) "We have not only increased the number of diseases, but we have also made them more dangerous and more fatal." (Rusch, 1906, 160)

Those who knew first-hand the short comings of drug therapy were the naturopaths. In the treatment of acute diseases, the naturopaths knew "that the ratio of recoveries from acute diseases [was] practically the same, irrespective of drugs and schools." (Juettner, 1906, 228) Those who pursued naturopathic practices found themselves treating allopathic patients who had been exposed to "a multitude of diagnostic errors and therapeutic sins." (Juettner, 1906, 228) With such diverging views, it is not surprising that the inconsistencies would play out in the realm of education and in the political arena.

What the "Medical Trust" was calling "medical science" was in this era increasingly informing the structure and mission of medical schools in America, especially after the Carnegie Commission published Flexner's report and the work of the General Education Fund began to affect medical school curriculum and facilities. During these formative years for the allopathic or biomedicine profession, MDs were driven by more questions than answers, burdened with more problems than solutions. For example, in their haste to monopolize the classification and diagnosis of disease and pathology generally, the early allopaths adopted some practices and methodologies that to this day we find less than helpful, often adversely affecting health and contributing only sporadically to prevention. The early naturopaths questioned the morality and ethics of some ramped up allopathic practices, such as vivisection and compulsory vaccination, against which "cruelties" *The Naturopath and Herald of Health* became a strong moral, public voice. As part of their questioning the value of vivisection, for example, the naturopaths asked, "Has anything been discovered that could have been discovered in no other way?" (Greene, 1904, 123)

Tensions of this kind between the increasingly heterodox Nature Cure doctors and the rapidly emerging orthodox allopathic medical system drifted into name slinging. The word 'quack' became commonplace as a derogatory label used by the allopaths to differentiate their expertise from their naturopathic competitors. Illustrative of this hostile relationship, the allopathic code of ethics published in 1905 evoked a clear stance:

We will have no professional intercourse with graduates of any other schools under any circumstances ... [and] in order to protect the public we must be ever ready to denounce as frauds and insane quacks any and all who through books and periodicals proclaim that our methods are mistaken. (The Ophtalmologist, 1905, 61-62)

In this mud-slinging landslide, the early naturopaths, who were so successful in applying water therapies and related nature-cure approaches, were viewed by the allopaths as "the water cure fakir" and as "another quack whose titles range from 'nature cure' to 'balneotechnic'. (S.A. B., 1905, 74)

State and federal medical laws were the next battleground. The allopathic medical societies were quite savvy about professional formation. They were extremely well funded in establishing the necessary legislative bills to elevate themselves to the position of enforcer of standards and protocols in primary care. The early naturopaths reacted to this growing wave of political maneuvering with outrage. They were increasingly alarmed, as Mann pointed out half a decade before Flexner, that "all medical laws that make the drug prescribers the protectors (?) of the public, and forbid the practice of other systems of therapy, are unconstitutional and should be repealed." (Mann, 1905, 159). In this rapidly shifting regulatory and public policy landscape, *The Medical Practice Act* took charge of determining the criteria for the legal right to practice medicine and naturopaths did not qualify. Subsequently, many naturopaths faced prosecution, jail time, heavy fines and persecution. One notable naturopath, Eugene Christian, was persecuted for practicing dietetics and prescribing raw food. "Because Mr. Christian and others have proven the incompetency of drug doctors by accepting cases that they have pronounced 'incurable' and curing them by scientific dieting, these doctors have been [hauled] to court as criminals." (Lust, 1907, 137) Ironically but significantly, the allopathic (or as it is known today, the 'biomedicine' profession) is beginning to assimilate nutrition into its domain, for example, as a modality to which MDs must now pay more attention, in its latest encroachment on natural medicine under the name, "integrative medicine". As recently as June 2013 the AMA declared that obesity, arising from the nutrition habits of Americans, is a "disease". (Miller, *New York Daily News*, June 19, 2013) Naturopathic doctors were raising the nutrition alarm a century ago, long before the era of high fructose corn syrup and hybridized wheat made a bad problem chronic.

In those early days, there was a coalition with varying strength between the naturopathic and osteopathic forces against the various newly formed "State Medical Boards". However, when osteopathy as a desired medical practice became acceptable to the A.M.A. (consistent with American osteopathy adopting biomedicine principles, philosophy and accreditation standards), the lines of commonality deteriorated between the naturopaths and the osteopaths. That convergence of American-style osteopathy into orthodox medicine had early manifestations. In California, for example, the legislature put into effect a new law regulating the practice of medicine on May 1st, 1907. "This law gave the osteopaths a place on the State board, together with the allopaths, homeopaths and eclectics." (*Los Angeles Times*, 1908, 29) The naturopaths were initially denied inclusion but with the indefatigable work of Dr. Carl Schultz and his wife, the practice of naturopathy in California was regulated for the first time March 14, 1907. However, the battle for dominance by the allopaths continued and it wasn't until the mid-1960s that the overt attack on the osteopaths by the A.M.A. abated.

Despite legislative changes, the prosecution of naturopaths continued and many succumbed. Dr Lust's journal was a venue to keep fellow naturopathic colleagues informed about who was arrested by the Medical Trusts. As an example, Dr. C. White, a California naturopath suffered under the new medical law, despite their 1907 inclusion. He notes: "during 16 years of drugless healing I have been arrested nine times and put under bonds, but I can truthfully say that there never has been any complaint filed by a patient, but in each case the arrest was caused and brought about by an MD." (White, 1908, 66) Another important case was brought against Dr. Carl Schultz himself for successfully treating a man and his wife "although they had been considered hopeless cases." (*Los Angeles Times*, 1908, 190) Back in the east, Bernarr Macfadden, the "well known editor of the *Physical Culture Magazine* and the champion of the physical culture movement in this country, was convicted for publishing articles and stories intended for better education and enlightenment." (Lust, 1908, 98) In the Pacific Northwest, another celebrated early naturopathic doctor," Dr. Linda Burfield Hazzard of Seattle, widely known as an advocate and practitioner of clinically appropriate fasting, [was] arrested [and] charged with willfully starving one of her patients to death. (Lust, 1911, 776)

We could surmise that the early Naturopaths were destined to follow on the heels of the Homeopaths who had been decimated in every way. In 1912, there were 173 homeopathic hospitals and numerous colleges in America. The largest, Milwaukee Orphan Asylum, was completely supported by endowment and contributions for its 2,125 bed hospital. Of those 173 hospitals, 30 ranged from the Milwaukee Orphan Asylum's 2,125 to at least 200 beds. The remaining 143 ranged from 195 beds to the smallest of the network at 30 beds, demonstrating the remarkable capacity of homeopathic care at that time. (Day et al., 1912, 160-172) Today, all of these homeopathic colleges and hospitals have been completely eradicated by the A.M.A's successful campaign to eliminate any competition in health care. Die or assimilate was the choice for the early 20th century homeopath. The naturopaths of that same era faced relentless discrimination by a medical profession who assumed political powers with a vengeance to make anyone quake in their presence.

Lust reports that he was "personally arrested 14 times and fined once $500 because a dirty woman sleuth of the Medical Trust with an unspeakable name took an electric light bath in my institution." (Lust, 1921, 480) The woman with the "unspeakable name" was Mrs. Francisca Bencecry who tried "for eight years continuously to get evidence against [Lust's] institution" (Lust, 1912, 391) and was successful. She was just one of the many that "the New York County Medical Society employed [as] spies, stool pigeons, sleuths, spittle lickers and hell servants to embarrass the Nature doctors." (Lust, 1921, 479) Lust explains further:

> The word 'Naturopath' was the magic word that set us free. Although being a misnomer, it covered the subject. It has come to stay as a living protest against the autocracy, coercion, imposition, intolerance and persecution of the New York County Medical Society Trust in particular, and the American Medical Association Trust in general. (Lust, 1921, 479)

The Medical Trust was not satisfied with the occupation of legislative seats; they had the goal of being America's "official medicine", including the United States military. In that regard, the Committee on Military Affairs on Sept 27, 1913 was responsible for enacting a law that authorized "two medical officers of the United States Army, with a rank of a captain and a major; two medical officers of the United States Navy, with a rank of lieutenant and lieutenant commander; and two medical officers of the United States Marine Hospital Corps, with a rank of lieutenant and lieutenant commander to a board to be known as the United States Medical Licensing Board." (Brandman, 1913, 723) By insinuating themselves into every possible location in American civic and military life, the MDs asserted their dominance.

The tension between the allopaths and the naturopaths heightened as more naturopaths were arrested and prosecuted for practicing medicine. As we survey the allopathic medical landscape today and see its exorbitant cost and its almost impenetrable power, the benefit of the historical record helps us to understand how that came about and to assess the experience of early naturopaths such as Erz who fought hard for *medical freedom*. Such developments made it clear to the early naturopaths that the medical laws were stacked against them, constituting as Erz claimed, "a mere farce as far as medical freedom and protection of the people are concerned." (Erz, 1912, 707) It was obvious that the "real object is to keep out competition and to persecute the drugless healer." (Erz, 1912, 707) Throughout this period, the naturopaths implored their readership, patients, [and] colleagues to fight medical monopoly and rally behind the political "candidates only who are for medical freedom." (Erz, 1912, 708)

In 1914, the Naturopathic profession advocated through *The Naturopath and Herald of Health* for the need for Naturopathic legislation to protect those practicing drugless therapies. From a baseline established in 1896 by the NY State Society of Naturopaths, there were some 500 drugless practitioners who were

> ... engaged in practice, using the so called natural methods of healing, such as hydrotherapy, light and air cure, diet, physical culture, Swedish movements and other systems of manipulation of the body. ... The underlying principle of these drugless methods of healing is prophylaxis or prevention of disease by right living and acquiring of normal habits, conforming to the laws of nature which underlie all things.(NY State Society of Naturopaths, 1914, 143)

The Society of Naturopaths documented extensively what they experienced as a ruthless and mercenary persecution by the Medical Trusts. These Trusts, the Society claimed, netted extensive funds and the means for New York County Medical Society, one of the "Trusts, to continue "actively the persecution of the drugless practitioners. Men and women who were guilty of no other offense than the giving of a bath or massage, the instruction in dietetics or systems of exercise, were heavily and unmercifully fined or sent to jail." (NY State Society of Naturopaths, 1914, 144) It was time for the New York Naturopaths to organize and establish the needed framework for their profession.

In an early widely distributed document called "Brief II", the early naturopaths identified the following methods of Naturopathy [as] "useful and indispensable":

DIETETICS
HYDROTHERAPY
PHYSICAL CULTURE
DYNAMIC BREATHING
MASSAGE
SWEDISH MOVEMENTS

STRUCTURAL ADJUSTMENT
SUN
LIGHT
AIR BATHS
KNEIPP CURE
JUST CURE
FASTING
(NY State Society of Naturopaths, 1914, 146)

The New York State Society of Naturopaths borrowed Henry Lind-lahr's definition of nature-cure [as] a "system of man-building harmonizing with the constructive principles of Nature, conforming to the physical, mental, moral and spiritual planes of being." (NY State Society of Naturopaths, 1914, 144)

Such "briefs" prepared by the New York Society of Naturopaths also laid down the first formal set of principles of naturopathy and proposed a philosophical platform of values which contributed to a sense of cohesion. Their early draft brief of principles has not metamorphosed much over this century; indeed, we can recognize the same principles that we have grown to acknowledge in our oaths today. In the bid for acceptance, the Society proclaimed:

NATUROPATHY, then, makes claim for recognition because:

• IT ENCOURAGES PERSONAL EFFORT AND SELFHOOD.

• IT SEEKS TO ADAPT ENVIRONMENT AND HABITS OF LIFE TO CONFORM TO NATURAL LAW.

• IT ASSISTS NATURE'S CLEANSING AND HEALING EFFORTS.

• ITS MEANS AND METHODS OF TREATMENT ARE HARMLESS, SIMPLE AND WITHIN EVERYBODY'S REACH.

• IT POINTS THE WAY TO A NATURAL METHOD OF LIVING AS REGARDS EATING, DRINKING, BREATHING, BATHING, DRESSING, WORKING, RESTING, THINKING, MORALITY.

(NY State Society of Naturopaths, 1914, 148)

Edward Earle Purinton was a prolific writer for the *Naturopath and Herald of Health.* In January 1915, he wrote for the profession a New Year's resolution: "our . . .first great need is to unite all the forces of drugless therapeutics under a single banner, with a single purpose, on a single method." (Purinton, 1915, 2) He describes the divide and discord among the drugless practitioners which were creating a climate of suffering in isolation. He called for a union of all drugless therapies and therapists, and encouraged his colleagues "to join the two or three national associations of hygienists and drugless physicians." (Purinton, 1915, 7)

Accordingly, by 1916 *The Naturopath and Herald of Health* underwent a new name change and became known as *Herald of Health and Naturopath.* However, the record does not indicate an announcement to let the readership know of this change nor did Lust leave any clues as to why he altered the wording in the name of his magazine.

In 1916, following Purinton's appeal to join forces, Lust published a similar letter in *Herald of Health and the Naturopath* rallying the naturopathic and drugless practitioners to create solidarity amongst all. He wrote, "in union is strength; in union we can break all the unconstitutional laws on the statute books in every state of the union; ... in union we can refuse submission to a mixed medical and osteopathic board, from whom we have never received a square deal in the past, now, nor [will] get it in the future." (Lust, 1916) Lust continued this entreaty:

> The American Naturopathic Association is not a family affair; not a one man's affair. It is an association which is made up of seventeen State Societies, six of them having their own State Charters and at the yearly convention the delegates of the different State Associations elect their officers for the National Organization. ... The practitioner will have a Society behind him that works for legislation, protection, defense ... the benefit of the Local and National Organization. (Lust, 1916)

This important history of drugless therapy was enriched by many other natural schools of healing. There was Wallace Fritz, for example, who recounts the history of the ancient Eclectic School of Medicine in 90 A.D. and traces the revival of the Eclectic Medical Institute of Cincinnati in 1845. (Fritz, 1916, 26) The Eclectic Medical Institute was founded on the proposition of maintaining "the utmost freedom of thought and investigation ... [and] to encourage the cultivation of Medical Science in a liberal spirit, especially in the development of resources of the vegetable Materia Medica, and the safest, speediest and most efficient methods of treating diseases." (Fritz, 1916, 27) Fritz includes a brief outline of the Thompsonians and their treatment rationale, a valuable element in the development of natural medicine in America.

These historical documents included not only detail about different groups and their influences, but also addressed controversial issues of the day, such as the question of compulsory vaccination. Anecdotal and quantitative information abound in these early writings. Lust, for example, wrote, "Any army doctor will tell you that innoculation with typhoid vaccine is made compulsory in the American Army. In the year 1912, this compulsory edict went into effect." (Lust, 1917, 256a) Statistics of military personnel dying from typhoid fever after having received the supposedly protective vaccine were strikingly high compared with those who were not vaccinated. Lust and his colleagues reported such data. "This fact stares us in the face that all those who were not vaccinated recovered." (Lust 1917, 256a)

As a case in point about the dichotomy between the allopaths and the naturopaths, the contentiousness of the vaccination question persists to this day. The naturopaths did not share the allopathic dogma of the germ theory. The allopathic doctor viewed the germs as the worst of the evils. Their solution was simple but Lindlahr questioned this logic: "kill the bug and cure the disease; that sounds plausible—but is it true?" (Lindlahr, 1910, 129) Lindlahr proposes, "Naturopathy holds that germs, bacteria and parasites are products of disease rather than its cause." (Lindlahr, 1910, 130) He continues, "Disease germs are present everywhere, on the food we eat, in the water we drink, in the air and dust we breathe, and on the money we handle." (Lindlahr, 1910, 130)

Lindlahr considered the naturopathic position against vaccinations as a crusade and weighed in on the dangers of vaccinations with comments such as: "When disease germs find in the human body the necessary conditions for growth and propagation—namely, lowered vitality, and their own congenial morbid soil—they multiply very rapidly and develop all the symptoms of that particular germ disease." (Lindlahr, 1910, 131) Vaccinations in the treatment of small pox developed in the body chronic forms of disease. (Lindlahr, 1910, 131) Lindlahr, if given the choice, would choose the acute expression of the disease above the chronic manifestations of a lowered vitality caused by the vaccinations.

The naturopaths were also pleased to document that so many women chose to pursue a naturopathic career. The presence of women in the profession is not, as some contemporary observers contend, a late twentieth century development. In his address to the 21st Annual American Naturopathic Association Convention, William Havard affirmed the contributions that women had made to the naturopathic profession. He maintained that "we have freely admitted women to our institutions. Our women are the bulwark of the present drugless profession. The biggest part the men are doing is talking; the women are doing the work. Healing, as a profession, is really a woman's work." (Havard, 1917, 330) Lust in his 1918 editorial concurs with Havard, "Our profession is a most noble one, and women are most admirably suited for it. The woman is a natural healer." (Lust, 1918, 709) Havard made a prescient statement: "You will never get anything from our present-day system of politics [male dominated]. You will never get the recognition you are looking for under existing conditions; you will have to wait until women come in, and come in strong." (Havard, 1917, 330)

Havard emphatically rallied his fellow naturopaths to be more involved in the strengthening of the profession, whatever their gender. In his article, *What does the A.N.A. Mean to You?*, he was imploring fellow colleagues to "labor as though you were the only one on whom responsibility rested, and this movement will grow." (Havard, 1918, 368) He confronts his colleagues with difficult questions, which seem alarmingly familiar today given the low per cent of membership in the current national body representing the profession. He asks, "The American Naturopathic Association commonly called the A.N.A. Now, what does it mean to you? Why are you in it—if you are?" (Havard, 1918, 368)

The topic of compulsory health insurance was brought up by Lust in a 1918 Editorial, *Social Health Insurance*. He asks, "How will this measure affect drugless physicians?" He knew very well that compulsory health insurance was positioned to cement allopathic medicine as the only medical choice. Those of us in practice today know how health insurance impacts the nature, momentum and autonomy of our livelihood. Lust continues, "There is not [the] slightest doubt but that if these measures now before several Legislatures are passed and become laws, it will bring the workingman more than ever under the autocratic control of the [allopathic] medical profession. ... The insured will be more likely to accept the [allopathic] medical benefits than if he were free to choose his favorite method of treatment." (Lust, 1918, 761)

Havard in his address to the 22nd Annual Convention of the A.N.A. lectured on yet another essential topic in this historical landscape, the business of healing. He had spent 8 months travelling across the country visiting naturopathic offices and after this trip he was disappointed that so many had "no ideals" and were more interested in the "business of healing ... [and] putting money in their pockets" (Havard, 1918, 764) than in the art and sacred trust of being a healer. Havard was a dedicated naturopath who revered the guiding principles of his profession. In this lecture he seems determined that his fellow colleagues see naturopathy as a high calling. He asks his colleagues, "If you are only patching up the conditions as they are, you are not really making the world any better. You are treating effects, not causes." (Havard, 1918, 765) He continues:

> Your real work should be educational. Educate the people into better ways of living and thinking, so that he next generation as it comes along will start out without the handicap of disease and disease suggestion, so that in time we may have here a wholesome, healthful nation of people, because it is only with that foundation

of a healthy body and a sound mind that we can hope to rise out of this false idea that we have, at present, regarding civilization. (Havard, 1918, 766)

As we have seen above, then, the Editorials of the *Herald of Health and Naturopath* were a venue for the journal to air grievances and claim victory. 1918 was an especially complex year, tragic in so many ways in the range of topics and concerns brought forward in their pages. The Spanish Flu, for example, was seen by many naturopathic doctors as a major determinant in ending WWI, a conflagration which had cost 9 million lives; however, the naturopathic community also noted that the endemic flu had killed an estimated 40 million people worldwide and need not have. The naturopaths were proud of their track record. Lust in his December, 1918 editorial with much pride, claimed:

> While our allopathic friends were futilely trying to check the "flu" with gauze masks, antiseptics, Dover's Powders and abundant food, and were wasting precious time trying to develop another poisonous serum from germs taken from the corpse of "flu" victims, the Naturopaths were achieving unrivalled successes. The death rate from pneumonia and influenza under Naturopathic treatment during the recent epidemic has been less than one percent. How does this compare with the 14 – 20% and even higher, under allopathic treatment? (Lust, 1918, 917-918)

The constraints placed on the early naturopaths by the 'regulars' forced them to adopt an oppositional viewpoint. Bernarr Macfadden voiced his repugnance strongly as he addressed his colleagues with the question, *"Shall We Have Medical Freedom?"* (Macfadden, 1919, 336) This question could easily be asked today as the naturopathic profession moves forward often too shyly among modern day 'regulars', grateful for recognition as an equal in the medical landscape, and suspicious of the hijacking of modalities in initiatives variously labeled "C.A.M." [complementary and alternative medicine] or "I.M." [Integrative Medicine]. We can count on our fingers the number of naturopaths who have been included at the federal and various health governmental tables,

places where decisions are taken and resources meted out for Medicare/
Medicaid and residency education. We simply have not reached equal-
ity and the A.M.A. attacks every state legislative effort with incomplete
information, inaccuracies and influence. We can, by understanding our
history, harken back a century to the time when early champions of natural medicine, such as Macfadden, argued, "It would appear that the
present control of all governmental policies concerned with the health
of the people by the representatives of allopathic medicine is a pure
usurpation of power without the consent of the people and without
representing the wishes of the people." (Macfadden, 1919, 336) The
pervasive nature of this "regulars" control on health care in America
in the early 20th century intensely irked many, including Benedict Lust.
He explains, "The greatest obstacle we have to contend with at present
is the obstinacy, the autocratic self-constituted control of the medical
combine, in other words, the medial imposition as it has fastened itself
upon the American people." (Lust, 1919, 438)

In a December, 1919 editorial, Wm. Havard hardly contains his
elation when reporting the triumph of the 23rd A.N.A. Convention.
Over 700 drugless physicians filled the convention hall to hear Dr. E. R.
Moras of Chicago and Dr. Wm. George of Columbus who, as Havard
reports, "... responded so handsomely to the appeal of Dr. Alzamon
Ira Lucas of Portland, Ore., for funds to found and erect the American Drugless University." (Havard, 1919, 583) Havard congratulated
these men for their unselfish generosity and reminded everyone of the
vision of Benedict Lust. He continued, "Be it remembered that [Dr. B.
Lust] is the one who has kept the altar fire burning through all these
years of discouragement. He has never lost faith even in the darkest
hours but has worked with single hearted purpose toward his objective." (Havard, 1919, 583)

While the Naturopaths were campaigning for their very own university, though, the Carnegie Foundation launched a number of projects
designed to give prominence to biomedicine. Not only did the General
Education Fund begin which would redesign undergraduate and professional graduate education, but special projects were launched. Lust

reported, "The Carnegie Corporation of New York has announced its purpose to give $5,000,000 for the use of the National Academy of Sciences and the National Research Council." (Lust, 1920, 61) Lust reminded everyone that the First World War "afforded a convincing demonstration of the dependence of modern nations upon scientific achievement, and nothing is more certain than that the United States will ultimately fall behind in its competition with the other great nations unless there be persistent and energetic effort expended to foster scientific research." (Lust, 1920, 61) Lust concluded with the lament, "think of how far we could carry our message with even half that sum when you consider what has already been done without a fund of any sort." (Lust, 1920, 62)

In the early 1900's there were many drugless therapists experiencing the same assault as the Naturopaths. Many of these professionals contributed their strong voices to the naturopathic publications because there was a growing commonality among the drugless therapist communities. In the beginning, the Naturopaths recognized the strength in solidarity. As Lust put it, the "naturopathic leaders have long cherished a fond dream – the union of all drugless factions into one great profession." (Lust, 1920, 269) In a July, 1920 editorial, Lust announced that it was time to "let the Osteopaths, the Chiropractors, the Mental Therapists and all the rest of the one-track systems go their own separate, independent ways." (Lust, 1920, 269) In helping these professions, he argued, "Naturopathy [had] actually compromised its position by encouraging the growth of these various systems." (Lust, 1920, 269) It was becoming very clear to the Naturopaths that the Osteopaths had been spared by the A.M.A. and that the Naturopaths were left in the cold.

During this period, too, not all was a bed of roses for the Chiropractors either; their profession experienced setbacks and obstacles, either in the form of irresponsible disinformation or more direct affronts in the form of injunctions generated by the medical profession. In Illinois, for example, Lust recounts, "Injunctions have been secured against fifty or more Chiropractors to prevent them from taking advantage of the protection offered by their Association. They dare not pay dues into the organization nor accept money or legal aid from the Association for fear of arrest for violation of the Illinois Medical Practice Act." Lust continues, "The plan was laid early in 1917 to eliminate the Chiropractor as a business competitor. Early in that year the Medical Doctors and Osteopaths of Illinois schemed to rob the already licensed drugless practitioners of the right to practice their respective arts obtained under the then existing Practice Act which was adequate and sufficient to meet all demands." (Lust, 1920, 321)

Given that the Osteopaths, Chiropractors and Naturopaths were on different paths, the A.N.A. recognized the necessity to "adopt some definite policy in dealing with other associations representing practitioners of different methods of drugless therapy and with individuals of these schools." (Lust, 1920, 373) At the A.N.A. 24th Annual Convention held in 1920, discussions occurred to "do the work nearest". This Convention was an effort to consolidate the "the fundamental principles of naturopathy" and "to determine what qualifications a Naturopath should possess". Lust called on his colleagues to recognize that a "wider publicity for our principles and methods" was needed as well as the serious consideration of "support of our schools and educational institutions". (Lust, 1920, 373-374)

One speaker at that same convention, Francesco Sanchelli, urged his colleagues that "steps be taken here and now for concerted action of all the drugless practitioners to the end that the public shall remain free" to choose the kind of health care that they want. (Sanchelli, 1920, 428) The convention was a supportive venue in which to recount for drugless practitioners current legislative events. Sanchelli informed his colleagues that, "seven separate bills [had] been introduced in the Senate and House of Representatives at Washington, proposing to establish a Federal Department of Health. These bills were drawn by, and are sponsored by, interests that have but one overwhelming ambition in life—to put all drugless practitioners out of business." (Sanchelli, 1920, 427)

As a backdrop to these legislative assaults and public relations confrontations, the allegation that diagnosis in naturopathic practice was sometimes being shunned by the Naturopaths contributed to claims that the N.D. could not be considered a primary care practitioner. An explanation purposed by Lust was that it was too easy to adopt someone's theory for disease which, his view, led to "laziness in making examinations." (Lust, 1921, 61) Another reason Lust includes by way of explaining this growing reluctance to communicate a diagnosis in the face of mounting allegations that the N.D. was practicing medicine without a license, was that the drugless physicians also were inclined to "rarely charge a sufficient fee for examination to warrant their spending the required amount of time to make a thorough diagnosis." (Lust, 1921, 61) Lust counseled his colleagues, "Find out everything you possibly can about the patient's condition: for remember your examination is not only made for the purpose of determining causes, but also the extent of the effects. ... Meet the medical man on his own ground and prove the superiority of your work." (Lust, 1921, 61-62)

Another persistent backdrop to these developments was the Flexner Report which documented the hodgepodge medical schools in America in the early 20th century. Lust assessed the spreading impact of Flexner's recommendations and of the work of the Carnegie and Rockefeller Foundations in financing a particular type of medical education. He wrote:

The American Medical Association—by this is meant more particularly the Inner Circle of paid officers and presidents of some of the larger schools—decided upon a classification of all medical schools. This arbitrary classification, let it be distinctly understood, was not governed by principles of worth, integrity or ideals, but by the sordid conditions of wealth, buildings, endowments, libraries, paid professors and affiliations with State Universities. (Lust, 1922, 111)

Lust was also not enamored by the emergence of 'the specialist'. He continues:

This may explain the phenomena of so many mentally astigmatic practitioners, who see in every patient a huge pathological ambulatory stomach, or a diseased heart, or whatever single organ of the body represents their particular specialty, and amenable only to their special treatment. (Lust, 1922, 112)

These pressures contributed to a most difficult time for the Naturopaths as they increasingly recognized that they were up against such powerful adversaries. Lust warned, "The Russell-Sage Foundation, the Carnegie foundation, and the Rockefeller Foundation are the chief bodies the American Medical Trust have made alliance with. From these sources they derive their greatest financial support in crippling schools not 'approved and accepted' according to the autocratic and sordid standards of the Inner Circle." (Lust, 1922, 112)

Among the naturopathic ranks, it is important to note, were Naturopaths who also had chiropractic training. This group was known as "the much abused class of Mixers." (Israel, 1923, 109) There were many Naturopaths and Chiropractors who felt that 'mixing' was not right. Palmer, the inventor of chiropractic, had a simple message to Mixers, "Either be a Chiropractor or a Naturopath. Be one or the other." (Israel, 1923, 109) Benjamin Israel, a Mixer, did not agree with Palmer's directive; by his own admission he thought more like a Naturopath. He goes on, "It has always been the policy of Naturopathy to include any Drugless science that gets some people well and so long as Naturopathy will remain broad and tolerant, its future policy will be the same." Israel then poses the question: "What crime is there when a Naturopathic physician takes a science that can do so much good for his patients and employs it in addition to his other Therapies?" (Israel, 1922, 110) He concludes his many arguments with, "instead of making chiropractic straight and sterile, make it efficient and worthwhile for the welfare of the sick." (Israel, 1922, 112)

Herbert Shelton, a true blue Naturopath, was not smitten, however, with the idea of the "Mixers" or with any collaboration. He states, "Naturopathy is older than Osteopathy, older than Chiropractic. Yet these ... are better known than is Naturopathy. Why is this?" (Shelton, 1923, 635) Not short on answers, he continues, "Naturopathy has been practiced under more names than any other system. At its birth it was christened the 'Water Cure'. Later it became known as 'Hydropathy', then 'Hygieo-therapy' and later 'Nature Cure'." (Shelton, 1923, 635) Shelton admits that the Naturopaths had been far too busy giving up "too much of our time and energy to helping the other schools to get before the public." (Shelton, 1923, 636)

In his view, the Naturopaths had "boosted Chiropractic" by including their articles in naturopathic journals. Shelton continues, "We have advertised these systems [Chiropractic, Osteopathy] and methods from their very beginning. We helped them on their feet; we helped popularize their methods and practice. We aided them in many ways." (Shelton, 1923, 636) And yet "today [1923], the Osteopath and the Chiropractor oppose us more than the medical men." (Shelton, 1923, 636-637) Shelton advocated that Naturopaths stay within their own kitchen and to "attend to our own business." (Shelton, 1923, 637)

As we can see, reviewing the broad spectrum of articles in the abundant literature of the period, the challenges to the professional formation of naturopathic medicine have been relentless. E. W. Cordingley perhaps captures an enduring challenge. In "*Let Us Standardize the Practice of Naturopathy*", he urges and rallies his colleagues to "agree on some common points and have … a certain positive regime that is at least in part applied to each and every patient." (Cordingley, 1923, 684) In this way, he insisted, patients will have "some common 'talking points' in explaining [Naturopathy] to their friends." (Cordingley, 1923, 684) The public could have a common understanding of what Naturopathy is and the "sooner it will become recognized as the greatest healing art the world has ever known." (Cordingley, 1923, 684) He was convinced that the medicine would endure. Cordingley had pursued practically every medical discipline including Chiropractic, Osteopathy, mechan-therapy, naprapathy, and even an MD license. He had experienced the merits and flaws and limitations of each, he said. His conclusion: "Naturopathy [is] the greatest healing art of all, because it takes from all whatever is good." (Cordingley, 1923, 685)

Cordingley viewed some forms of manipulative therapy and dietary counsel as core treatments for each patient that would come to unifying a standardized Naturopathic treatment which all patients could come to expect from any Naturopath that they visited. "Of course, we know that no two patients should be treated exactly alike." (Cordingley, 1923, 684) So he advised, "To select your adjunct treatment to fit the particular case." (Cordingley, 1923, 686) He understood the power and enduring value of the patient-centered nature of naturopathic medicine, an understanding of primary care which endures to this day as an ideal. Even the allopaths with their "integrative medicine" efforts know this.

Contemporary Naturopathic doctors would do well to remember Cordingley's insistence that every Naturopath's duty was to join his or her National Association. He left us a prophetic claim, that "ten years from now we are going to see 'Naturopath' signs in every city of any importance in the United States, and the practitioner will be proud to be able to call himself a Naturopath, because it will mean that he is a member of the most progressive and most successful healing system in the world." (Cordingley, 1923, 686)

Sussanna Czeranko, ND, BBE

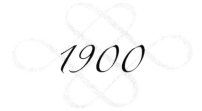

A Brief History Of Natural Healing
Benedict Lust

Allopathy
Friedrich Eduard Bilz

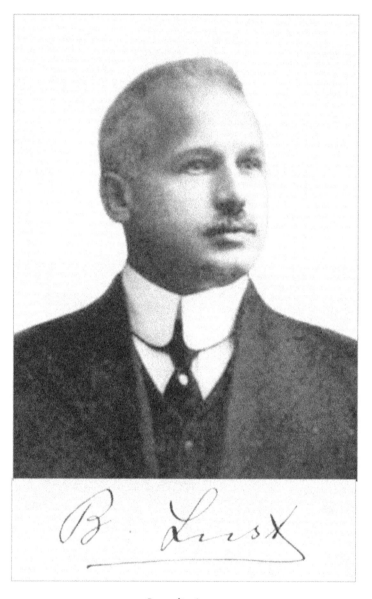

Benedict Lust.

A Brief History Of Natural Healing

by Benedict Lust

The Kneipp Water Cure Monthly I(1), 2-5. (1900)

Long, long ago, in those old times of which history tells a sort of fairytale, when people were not so mightily learned and the learned did not pretend to be so much wiser than the creator, in those times we already heard about people who advocated the study of nature's laws and proved to suffering humanity how easy it is to become healthy and well by nature's simple remedies.

The bath predominated to such an extent in those days that in some countries the bath was a part of religious functions.

The first authentic proof of the application of a sort of water-cure comes from ancient Rome. About the time Christ was borne in Palestine, there lived in ancient Rome a former slave named Antonius Musa, who practiced a water-cure and was so well known for his great success that emperor Augustus and his friend Horatius called upon him for help and cure. These two worthy gentlemen who had imbibed too freely of the heavy wines sunny Italy produces. The medical authorities of ancient Rome tried in vain to cure the imperator and his friend.

What the learned doctors could not do in a very long time was done by the former slave in a comparatively short time. The water-cure soon became a means of strengthening the systems of all those who had ruined their health by living too high. The example of the great Augustus was followed by thousands with good results.

But already about 400 B.C. Hippokrates [sic] tells us that cold water was considered one of the best remedies for quite a number of ailments. His statements were corroborated by Galenus in Pergamus (died about 200 A.D.) and Asklepiades on the island of Samos.

Up to Hippokrates no medical science existed. Hippokrates was the first to classify all medical experiences and is consequently the originator and founder of medical science. But little or nothing was done to cultivate the seed during more than one thousand years, till Theophrastus Paracelsus (who died September 23, 1541) surprised the world by his statement: *Natura artis magistra*, in plain English: Nature is art's teacher.

Again more than 200 years had to roll by till the water-cure was made a regular study, till I.S. Hahn, a physician in Schweidnitz (died 1773), wrote his pamphlet defending the water-cure and announced, that in the future he would follow its principles. After Hahn we find Samuel Hahnemann as an apostle of the water-cure in 1784. Slow progress was made in the eighteenth century and not much was done during the first two decades of the 19th century. It was not till 1826 that the agitation became more lively and not till Vincenz Priessnitz opened the first water-cure sanitarium in Graefenberg in Austrian Silesia, that interests in this new mode of healing became more general.

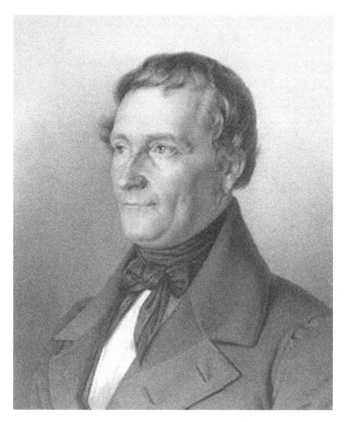

Vincenz Priessnitz, Founder of The Water Cure.

VINCENZ PRIESSNITZ

Vincenz Priessnitz was born on October 4, 1799 in Graefenberg. He was the son of a poor blind farmer and early, when other children spent their time playing, young Vincenz had to look after his father's little farm. The old saying became true again. Experience is the best teacher. Not Professors who cut up living beings in the dark ill smelling schoolrooms, in order to give their pupils an idea of nature's masterhand, were his teachers, but nature itself was his guide and mentor. He observed nature and knew how to use the results of his observations for the best and welfare of his fellow-beings. Of course from the beginning his system was not all perfection. He improved on it all the time. Physicians from all parts of Europe came to Graefenberg to study his water-cure, but Priessnitz was not very fond of these learned pupils. Referring to these gentlemen, he said one day: "They are the worst of all, to become good followers of my principles they have to forget too much. Should my sanitarium fall into the hands of a physician after my death, it will be ruined in a very short time." The principle mistake, made by these physicians, was the way they studied the water-cure. They inquired for instance, how long, how deep and how wide the bath-tubs were, or took the measure of the bandages used without accepting any other explanation, for these learned gentlemen knew everything. They were under the impression that their diplomas covered the ground, and they as licensed dispensers of health *ergo ipso facto* understood everything about it. But these learned pupils of Priessnitz did not have much success with their patients, for they applied water in the same way they applied drugs; they bothered too much with the art of it and paid too little attention to the nature of the water cure and the patient. In 1851 Josef Schindler became the successor of Vincenz Priessnitz, who died November 28th in the same year. Thousands have to thank Schindler for their health and among them the Duke of Nassau and the Grandduke of Mecklenburg who was given up by his physicians, but after a short stay left Graefenberg as a healthy man. The Grandduke was so much pleased that he sent four physicians to Graefenberg every year to study the water-cure. In August 1888 King Karol I. of Rumania also was a guest in Graefenberg.

Priessnitz' principles are best represented by the following statement of his own: "Not the cold but the heat produced by the cold water
is the healing factor."

JOHANN SCHROTH

At the same time, in the same neighborhood in Austrian Silesia
and under the same financial circumstances the other great apostle of
natural healing and contemporary of Priessnitz was born and brought
up. He was Johann Schroth, born February 11, 1798. Priessnitz and
Schroth were schoolmates in Freiwaldau. When little Johann reached
the age of seven, his father who had been a farmer like Priessnitz' father,
died. Schroth's mother married again after a short time and the time
for work had come for him. But Johann became a faithful worker in
the interest of the family, indeed so faithful that his stepfather decided
to leave the farm to him, instead of leaving it to his own sons. Besides
his farm Schroth established a livery stable and express business and
became well to do. The express business was destined to turn his mind
to natural healing. In 1817 a horse broke Schroth's kneecap and knee-
bones. A healing was accomplished but was so imperfect that Schroth
could not bend his leg and had to go lame.

In those times the expressman was a very important factor in commerce, for other means of communication were scarce. It was cus-
tom in those days that the expressman walked by his wagon, but on
account of his lame leg Schroth could not follow it and had to sit on his
wagon. In one of his travels he met a monk who taking him for lazy
reprimanded him severely. After Schroth had told him about his leg,
the monk gave him the advice, to wash his knee with cold water several
times a day. Schroth could not do that, but thought that a piece of wet
heavy cloth, covered by a piece of dry cloth would do just as well and
could be left around the knee for a long time. In fact he left this heavy
bandage on the knee for hours until it became quite dry. During the
night he used more water and a still heavier cloth and wrapped the leg
in a woolen blanket. The effect was wonderful. The swelling disappeared, the veins again became soft and after ten weeks treatment the

former stiff leg was as well as the other one. Nobody could tell which leg was once the sore one.

This cure and its results formed the foundation on which Johann Schroth built his system, which we perfected more and more. At first he only applied wet bandages in cases of wounds, callosity, contusions and stiffness of joints etc., etc. In all cases the greatest success followed. This encouraged Schroth to try his system in cases of sickness of interior organs. He valued wet heat very much for this reason. He observed that the corn to grow needed moisture and heat, but not too much of either, therefore he considered wet heat as the main condition of the origin and the maintenance of all organic creations (men, animals and plants). At the same time he was convinced that the lack of wet heat would produce sickness and that the application of wet heat would sure sickness.

To Schroth principally the merit is due to proving the importance of a well regulated diet in all cases of sickness. His great gift of observing every detail in every case brought his system to a very high standard of perfection. He found that a fever often produced good results and even was necessary to secrete morbid matter. He succeeded in chronic cases to bring about the state of fever which served to secrete this morbid matter, he succeeded in regulating this fever till the system was free of sickness. We cite one instance to show how Schroth used this gift of observing all details and points offered to him by chance and making use of them for the benefit of suffering humanity.

While in the express business he often stopped in a roadhouse, whose host was very fat, so fat indeed that it was a great trouble for him to move. This man used to sit in his chair all day, never got up to serve his customers, but called one of his men to perform this duty. Schroth had not seen this man for some time and was very much astonished to find his host jump up the next time he entered. But how the man had changed! All the fat had disappeared, the man was as thin as thin could be and moved about as easy as anybody. Of course Schroth was surprised and had to get an explanation. Trouble in his family had brought the host on the verge of bankruptcy. Instead of the life of comfort and ease, he had to work and got sorrow in the bargain. That big mass of fat which that man had in his body could only have left it by secretion. The excitement, his troubles, the change in his diet after having lost his money had been the means, by which the result was obtained. Schroth knew how to use these points and in many a case he succeeded to reduce the weight of a patient by only changing his diet and giving him the necessary excitement to produce a sort of fever which secreted all the morbid matter and fat.

The natural organs of secretion are bowels, kidneys, skin and lungs. Stool, water, perspiration and sputum are the natural results of secreting all superfluous matter. A good healthy stomach, well working bowels and kidneys etc., etc., are essential for obtaining good results, therefore, Schroth put all his energies and knowledge to strengthening and cleansing these organs. Good pure food and a good digestion can only produce good chyle, but good chyle must by degrees overcome all morbid matter. Nature's power of healing must be assisted and the battle is half won. Nature will do the rest. Schroth assisted nature by creating wet heat and by regulating the diet of the patient according to his case.

Schroth's system of dietetical healing was a success. One of his greatest cures was the healing of Duke William of Wurttemberg who as captain in an Austrian regiment was wounded one inch under the right knee in the battle of Novarra, March 28, 1849. For eight months physicians tried in vain to heal the wound which grew worse and worse until Schroth undertook the healing. In sixteen weeks the prince was as well as before the battle of Novarra and so delighted, that he recommended Schroth's system to all his comrades suffering from old or new wounds.

Johann Schroth died March 26, 1856.

Hippokrates, Antonius Musa, Theophrastus Paracelsus, I.S. Hahn, Samuel Hahnemann, Vincenz Priessnitz and Johann Schroth laid the foundations for a system of healing in which cold water is the factor to produce natural wet heat and natural wet heat is therefore the real factor to secrete morbid matter and to produce health. From 400 B.C.

up to to-day this science of natural healing advanced constantly, but no man gained greater fame and was more successful than Sebastian Kneipp, the priest and benefactor of mankind. Like all his predecessors Kneipp gained his knowledge by his own experience, Kneipp was chosen by providence to deliver to men a message of truth and to fulfill a sacred mission on earth.

SEBASTIAN KNEIPP

Sebastian Kneipp too was the son of poor and humble parents. He was born in an obscure, small Bavarian country place named Ottobeuren. His father was a weaver and had trouble enough to earn sufficient money to keep his little family from actual starvation. Consequently young Sebastian early became acquainted with the hardships and miseries of life. There was something unusual however, about him. "He was not at all like the rest," is the description of one of his playmates, "he was always buried in his books or was singing glorias, clever he was also."

The miserable and poor surroundings in which he had to pass his youth apparently doomed young Kneipp to the life of a journeyman weaver and nobody dreamed at that time that the plain, poor country lad, with absolutely no opportunities to acquire even a limited education, was yet to distinguish himself in life and to gain an international reputation. It is more than likely that is he had found the struggle easier and success less troublesome he would not have become of such great benefit to the world.

As soon as Sebastian Kneipp began to think for himself, he became ambitious to study for the priesthood. Neither he nor his parents could see the slightest chance for realizing his dreams. Kneipp did not despair, he believed in his destiny, he worked hard to gain his point and he succeeded. This belief in himself, this belief in his own qualities and abilities, this iron will to be of greater service to humanity than as a simple journeyman weaver gave the strength to him to overcome all difficulties. He was moved by no mean or selfish motive. He was not hunting the dollar or struggled to better his position. He never thought of improving his financial conditions. His only aim was to be of service to his fellowmen. From the first moment the idea entered his brains he worked hard to realize his dream and become a priest, but not before he was well advanced in the twenties he succeeded in interesting a curate in his plan. This good-hearted priest gave him his first mental training and educated the young weaver until he could enter college. In college Kneipp worked with so much earnestness and zeal that his weak body collapsed under the strain. For the next two years Kneipp was treated by a benevolent physician with bad results. He came pretty near abandoning his plan, when by chance a book, treating of the water-cure, fell into his hands. He read and read and read and when he was through reading his mind was filled with joy. New hope had moved into his heart. What the good doctor could not do, he knew, he would do. Kneipp tried the water-cure on his own body and in a very short time not only was he able to take up again and finish his studies but he became stronger and healthier than ever before. From the moment his health was restored, Kneipp made the water-cure his special study and soon became an expert in all matters pertaining to it.

To Kneipp principally the merit is due of calling the attention of suffering humanity to the healing properties of some herbs. He tested the nourishing qualities of different kinds of food, he tested the different kinds of materials used to protect the body against the direct influence of the temperature of the air and succeeded in building up a system of healing which has brought health and with it happiness into many a home, where the two were not known before for a long time.

Kneipp's system is as simple as his success is great; Kneipp defended the principle that all origin of disease was in the blood, containing either morbid matter or not circulating right. The influence of cold water was to regulate the circulation of the blood and to force it to secrete morbid matter by means of the skin. Small-pox and typhoid fever for instance he cured in comparatively a short time. Space does not permit us to name all the diseases which Kneipp cured successfully, but there is hardly a case in which he was not successful and which cannot be cured by his method. It strengthens and hardens the whole human system.

Kneipp never treated one part of the body only, but always the whole organism of the patient.

Kneipp's method is light and reasonable. Cold water is used and used with care. The patient is never treated for more than from one to three minutes, often seconds are sufficient. After treatment no towel is used, but heat is produced by exercise, if possible in the open air. A patient who is too weak for exercise has to get warm in bed and soon feels comfortable.

Kneipp's own discovery is the healing power of the gush or pour. The Kneipp pours strengthen the nerves and muscles and in this way effect a general change in the whole organism. The action of the respiratory organs, the action of the organs of secretion, the circulation of the blood as well as metabolic assimilation are powerfully stirred up. The pours or gushes take up very little time but their beneficial effect is great.

Kneipp's diet is simple and nourishing. His strength-giving soups, his Kneipp-bread and his malt-coffee are foods, which are used by the many thousands who follow his principles of a simple and natural mode of living.

The next century will give him and his system full credit, millions will benefit from his teachings, mountains of pain and sorrow will be removed by his pours. Sebastian Kneipp, the modest priest of that little Bavarian village Woerishofen, was indeed God's messenger of glad tidings and good health.

The water-cure became a science, not a science taught by Professors in Highschools, but the science of healing of the plain and poor people. Soon there was a change though. The rich man noticed that the poor man not only got more for his money, but something which was far better in quality. The rich man, of course, was relieved from pain by his physician, but very soon he had to consult the doctor, the man of medical science, again and again. The drugs stopped one pain, on ailment, only to produce another one. How different was the result of the poor man's treatment! He was not only relieved from pain without the use of drugs, but his system was improved and cleansed, he felt better, he was stronger and the best of all by following the simple rules of natural healing he began to forget altogether that bodily pains existed. These simple rules not only produced health, but enabled their followers to keep their bodies in good health always. Health, long life and naturally happiness were gained by a natural treatment of ailment and sickness.

This great success called the attention of all the world to the natural systems of healing. Men of brains and understanding, men who felt it a duty to help suffering humanity and to enlighten the world, took up the study of this new science. Physicians even commenced to recognize the value and importance of a natural and drugless system of healing. These men studied nature's means for treating ailments and sickness. Next to water and air, electricity and magnetism became factors in the forms of treatment.

ARNOLD RIKLI

Arnold Rikli was the first to call the attention of the world to the value of the light-, air-, and sun-bath. Rikli was born February 13th, 1823. As a boy he had occasion to become acquainted with these light-, air-, and sun-baths and experience was his only teacher. He tried the effects of these baths on his own body and was convinced that they would become a great factor in the art of natural healing. A master never falls from heaven and years of earnest study were necessary to perfect his system.

What is light-, air-, and sun-bath, our readers will ask. That is easy to explain. The naked body is exposed in the open air to the influence of light and sunheat. What is the effect of such a bath, may be the next question. Light is absorbed by the skin and invigorates the system, it is a necessity to the maintenance of human or animal life, it accelerates metabolic assimilation and increases the secretion of carbonaceous matter.

Light darkens the skin and makes it anaesthetic. There is casual coherence between the light of the sun and the development of all

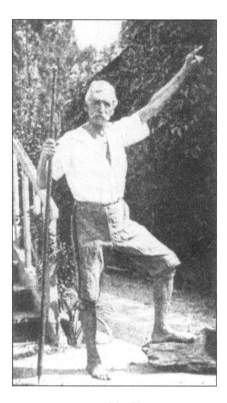

Arnold Rikli.

organic life. To Rikli principally the merit is due of proving the influence of light upon the nerves, metabolic assimilation, nutrition, sanguification and the organism in general. Not in the dark but under the influence of the light of the sun only life can take its natural course; men need light and air. It was Rikli who started the theory that men are born naked, that it was their designation to live like moving plants in the ocean of light and air. Rikli was the first to show the influence and the effect of light, air and water upon the human organism and to make use of the healing qualities of them.

Of course, Rikli had his troubles. He was taken for crazy by the majority, but his theories found followers, who practised them with beneficial results. There are quite a number of sanitariums in Europe to-day, in which the light-air-baths are the principal means of treating certain ailments.

There is no doubt, the systems of natural healing will form the foundation of the medical science of the next century. The great physician of to-day are very well aware of the fact that drugs don't cure, as the celebrated Professor Dr. med. Wunderlich said: "We have to be thankful to every shepherd and every old woman for a remedy against sickness, for we have none."

The science of natural healing has spread like wild-fire. In every country there are followers of the different systems and methods. Thousands are treated with good results and among these thousands are a very large percentage who were given up as uncurable by the physicians of the old school. In the United States also the water-cure and kindred branches of natural healing have got many followers and friends. People feel that a change is necessary. When the first followers of the principles of our great master Kneipp practised one of his rules, the walking in the grass wet with morning dew, people thought them crazy and to-day the majority believe that taking the Kneipp-cure means walking in the grass.

By degrees this misunderstanding disappears. The great cures which practitioners of all branches of natural healing have accomplished have changed many minds, and to-day there are a large number of sanitariums throughout the country, where patients are treated without drugs according to nature's laws.

> *Kneipp's system is as simple as his success is great; Kneipp defended the principle that all origin of disease was in the blood, containing either morbid matter or not circulating right. The influence of cold water was the regulate the circulation of the blood and to force it to secrete morbid matter by means of the skin. Small-pox and typhoid fever for instance he cured in comparatively a short time.*

Allopathy

by Friedrich Eduard Bilz

The Kneipp Water-Cure Monthly, I(7), 125. (1900)

Allopathy is that system of treatment, which tries to affect by medicine the reversal of the symptoms characterizing a disease. (Medical men are the votaries of this system.) It looks upon the symptoms of a disease as errors of nature, and endeavors to remove them by chemical means, not considering that in doing so the whole of the organic system gets disturbed and weakened in the performance of its functions - nay, is often entirely crippled. Allopathy tries to kill pain temporarily by narcotics, to great injury of the nerves or sensation, which, if anything, get paralyzed by the employment of such palliatives. It attempts to produce sleep by the aid of morphia and chloral hydrate, thus weakening the central nervous system and prolonging illness, or, if the patient has but small powers of resistance, sending him to the realms of eternal rest. Allopathy suppresses the troublesome cough, meant by nature to eject for the patient's benefit the gathering secretions of the respiratory organs. Allopathy relieves the rectum of accumulated masses of excrement by injurious purgatives, independent of the fact that such remedies overstimulate the nerves of the rectum, thus causing the whole muscular system of that part to lose its needful elasticity. In the same way it arrests the process of fermentation in cases of diarrhea arising from congestion of the rectum with fermenting matter, in doing which the greatest injury may be caused to the system. Allopathy busts of annihilating all fermenting substances, such as bacteria, bacilli, etc., by chemicals—i.e., casting out the devil by Beelzebub. But besides bacilli, bacteria, etc., healthy tissues are destroyed at the same time, and not only is the morbid matter not secreted, but it is joined by medical poisons, and these combined greatly impede nature in its efforts to purify itself. Fever—the very spirit of nature's endeavor to help herself— allopathy suppresses with poisons, which, having entered the system, are at once rendered harmless, as far as can be effected by the vital power. But in these efforts of nature a great amount of strength, and therefore heat (strength is heat) is lost. Still, what more is wanted? The result aimed at, viz.: subduing the fever is attained. A sadly fallacious result.

Want of space renders us unable to expose in this article the entire unreality of allopathy as a therapeutic agent. This much may be said- that we give proof positive in this work by practically tested advice, and independent of any theory, that disease can be cured without inju- rious medicines, which are at the best questionable as to their results. We wish the reader, by perusing this work, to gain the firm conviction that the application of allopathy cannot but be harmful in every case.

We have now only to explain why the so-called scientific physician clings so obstinately to allopathy. Prof. Gustav Jaeger does so by quot- ing the saying: "The more versed, the more perverse." The influence exerted by pedantry more or less on every practical science, particu- larly on therapeutics, is notoriously a baneful one, as was very strik- ingly demonstrated to the world in the case of the late German Emperor Frederick. What that influence means is easily explained. Pedantry, as it is cultivated at the higher clinical colleges, proceeds in the following manner: A dictum, or an enemy nothing, is pronounced; this dictum or this nothing is then surrounded by all kinds of thorny "ifs" and "buts," consideration, subterfuges, sophisms, pros and cons, etc. The medical student is then placed within the thorny hedge thus formed, and he is perfectly safe there; nothing can spirit him away; nobody can get at him. To every fact, to every opinion he opposes his "ifs" and his "buts"; he is perfectly proof against all advice, and, being as a rule, unable to get through this hedge, he is hopelessly lost.

With the release of higher therapeutics from the trammels of ped- antry, half the work, but not more than half the work, has been done. (Bilz *Natural Healing*)

> *It looks upon the symptoms of a disease as errors of nature, and endeavors to remove them by chemical means, not considering that in doing so the whole of the organic system gets disturbed and weakened in the performance of its functions—nay, is often entirely crippled.*

1901

Christian Science And Naturopathy
Ludwig Staden, Naturopathic Physician

———

"Key" Or "How To Obtain Long Life"
John F. Morgan

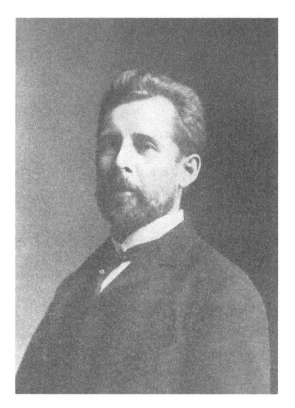
Ludwig Staden, Naturopathic Physician.

CHRISTIAN SCIENCE AND NATUROPATHY

by Ludwig Staden, Naturopathic Physician

The Kneipp Water-Cure Monthly, II(4), 100. (1901)

There is much talk about Christian Science; everybody nowadays knows what this Science means. Medical Science is fighting it wherever there is a chance. If a Christian Science healer loses a
patient the daily papers inform the public immediately, not forgetting
the commentaries concerning the absurdity and craziness of such healers; sometimes they even recommend putting such healers into prison.
Of the thousands who daily die under medical treatment they never
mention one word. The public are talking, according to the papers.
This is no wonder, as the great masses never use their own judgment,
and so Christian Science is mostly condemned just like Naturopathy.

There is no doubt that Christian Science is a good thing, if in the
hands of healers who are honest and true. If Christ is the Saviour, why
do not the Christ-thoughts save, and if they do not, of what possible
good are they? says Rev. Francis Mason. This is a fine question and I
liked to hear it answered by empiric science. Christian Science in itself
is a truth. It must be a truth, but it is an old truth and not a new science,
as Mrs. Eddy, the founder of Christian Science, pretends. It is an old,
old truth and can be traced far back to the Vedas. Mrs. Eddy and her
adherents are mistaken in teaching that Christian Science and nothing
else is the only method of healing. There is in fact no method of healing
that can make such a claim, as the power of healing is not without, but
within everybody. It is an individual power and therefore everybody
can heal and has a right to heal, if he understands and realizes this
power, if he can awaken it, or is able to perceive it.

Christian Scientists further make the mistake in pretending that the
body does not exist; only the soul if there is no body, and if there is no
disease, why do they heal at all? If disease does not exist, there need be
no healing and there need not be any method of healing. Who in the
world can pretend the non-existence of the body or of matter? Matter

is just as much unknown as the spirit; Science only knows the change of matter, but never matter itself, and never will know it. Indeed all human life taken from a divine standpoint is a folly, because human existence exists and as the soul never can be sick, consequently they deny any disease. This is a great contradiction; nothing else but the result of non-perception or, we may say, of ignorance. Taken from a human standpoint all human life, all our doing and being is a necessity, because even surrounded by illusions and being an illusion himself man has to yield to the conditions of such an illusory existence. And this is the reason why we must recognize the body and consequently we cannot help yielding to the circumstances under which this body exists. Naturopathy will never deny the great truth of the healing power of the Christ-thought, but will also give credit to other healing factors taken from nature, and this will make Naturopathy superior to Christian Science. I do not see any reason why we should not apply to a fever patient a cool sponge bath or a cool half bath or a wet pack, etc.; what an immense relief to such a patient is such a treatment; the physiological effect is in the finest harmony with the physiological functions of the human organism.

I can see all material things with my physical eye, and if I close it or if I am blind I cannot see the world; do you doubt it? But I can see many things which I cannot see with my physical eye which I only can see with my spiritual eye; why should I wish to see only one world and not the other? There is medical science that sees only the physical and there is Christian mental science in regard to external things would be based on mere speculation, if we had not the capacity of seeing external phenomena, so also the highest science must be mere speculation in regard to spiritual things for those who have no spiritual perception. But who has the spiritual and physical perception for whom there is no more doubt, and this is expressed in the Bible by the words: "Pray and work."

Ludwig Staden
Naturopathic Physician,
336 Schermerhorn St., Brooklyn

"Key" or "How to Obtain Long Life"

by John F. Morgan

Quotes from The Kneipp Water Cure Monthly, II(6), 149-50. (1901)

Medical Freedom

A man ought to be as free to select his physician as his black-smith, for he alone is to profit or suffer by his choice. The responsibility is his.

—*Wm. E. Gladstone*

How is it that there are a thousand ways in which I may be permitted to damn my soul, but when it comes to a trivial matter like temporary ill health, the Legislature must prescribe how I shall do it. It is absurd and ridiculous."

—*Mark Twain*

Medical Monopoly

I think it would be better for the profession if we all would recognize the fact, that it is better to have patients to die under scientific treatment, than to recover under empirical treatment, therefore use tonics if needed for your dignity and thereby accept no dictating by the laity.

—B. F. Posy, M.D.

Medical Times, Philadelphia, Pa. and Boston, Mass., Oct., 1900

Consequently we cannot help yielding to the circumstances under which this body exists. Naturopathy will never deny the great truth of the healing power of the Christ-thought, but will also give credit to other healing factors taken from nature, and this will make Naturopathy superior to Christian Science.

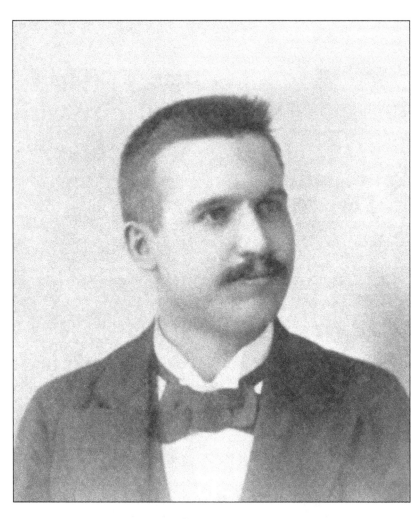

Benedict Lust in 1902.

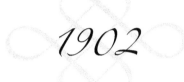

1902

A Happy New Year!
Benedict Lust

———

Editorial Drift
Benedict Lust

THE NATUROPATH

... AND ...

DEVOTED TO
NATUROPATHY:
THE SCIENCE
OF PHYSICAL
AND MENTAL
REGENERATION

HERALD OF HEALTH

FORMERLY

THE KNEIPP WATER CURE MONTHLY

PUBLISHED
MONTHLY
IN ENGLISH
AND GERMAN

SUBSCRIPTION:
$1.00 A YEAR IN ADVANCE,
WITH FOREIGN POSTAGE $1.50
SINGLE COPIES 10 CTS.

BENEDICT LUST, EDITOR AND PROPRIETOR,

111 EAST 59TH STREET, NEW YORK, U. S. A.

ESTABLISHED 1896.

Vol. III   No. 1   JANUARY, 1902   Whole No. 25

Masthead, first issue of *The Naturopath and Herald of Health,* January 1902.

A Happy New Year!

by Benedict Lust

The Naturopath and Herald of Health, III(1), 13-14. (1902)

To all our readers, patrons and well-wishers.
We look back with pride to the past two years, and may well be satisfied with the progress achieved by our magazines.

Our German publication, *Amerikanische Kneipp-Blätter*, will begin its seventh year with its January issue, and, although it had to overcome a great many difficulties at first, it has gradually worked its way into recognition as one of the leading hygienic magazines published in this country in the German language.

Its sister-publication, *The American Kneipp-Water Cure Monthly*, has also had to fight its way into the ranks of the hygienic standard monthlies. It had a very arduous task before it in attempting to call the attention of the great American reading public to its existence. As soon as any lady or gentleman reader had glanced through one of our monthly issues, our magazine and its efforts were highly appreciated.

But there was one very great impediment which hampered the *Kneipp-Water Cure Monthly* from growing with rapidity; this was its name.

The name of the esteemed late very Rev. Sebastian Kneipp, who preached and practiced the water-cure treatment for so many years in Woerishofen in Germany, is a well-known name in German circles—but not so amongst the Americans.

Most of the average American readers associate the name of "Kneipp" with the "fad" of walking barefoot (in the grass). They are quite right! Kneipp did advise a number of his patients to walk barefoot, but this does not mean to say that this is the entire and complete Kneipp cure. Not by any means! The late Rev. Seb. Kneipp wrote four valuable books which were published in German before his demise. These are: *My Water-Cure* (The Kneipp Cure), *Thus Shalt Thou Live*, *My Will*, and Codicil to *My Will*.

These books were found to be so exceedingly valuable that they were translated into almost every known language.*

When we started to publish our American *Kneipp Water Cure Monthly*, we had unfortunately forgotten to consider the important point that Kneipp was almost unknown in American reading circles. But we very soon found out what up-hill work we had before us when the subscriptions were coming in very slowly only. Advertisers also generally objected to the name, and we decided to give our American publication the right and correct name, viz., *The Naturopath and Herald of Health*.

What is Naturopathy? will naturally be now asked by every one. Naturopathy embodies all natural healing methods, including Hydrotherapy (Priessnitz, Kneipp and Just's systems), Osteopathy, Heliotherapy (sun, light, and air cure), Hygienic and Physical and Mental Culture to the exclusion of all drugs and non-accidental surgery.

The *Naturopath*, as is implied by its name, will endeavor to place before the American reading public, in subsequent essays and contributions by various well-known writers, the quintessence of natural hygiene. This Naturopathic magazine will not accept any obnoxious or quack advertisements. No patent-medicines nor poisonous drugs of any kind compounded in chemical laboratories will be admitted in our columns, and the general tenure of the contents of each month's issue will be not only instructive but also agreeable reading. Of course a magazine of this kind has to rely solely on the support and assistance of its patrons and well-wishers. We will always highly appreciate short contributions sent in by any of our readers having reference to any of the subjects discussed in our magazine, and will cheerfully mail free sample copies to any number of names sent us.

Our readers of the fair and gentle sex especially, by distributing our magazines or calling attention to the same, will benefit our cause to a very great extent. Many a young man, if his attention would only be called to our magazine by the lips of some sweet womanly woman, would not only peruse its pages with attention, but also be won over to our cause with much greater certainty than if he were guided by chance only to glance through one of our sample copies.

May we therefore hope that our numerous patrons, readers, advertisers and well-wishers will bestow upon our undertaking the kind patronage it so richly deserves, and may we hope that they will not obliterate from their memory the embodiment of all natural healing methods: "Naturopathy."

* They are for sale at nearly every bookstore in the United States, and if not producible, we will be pleased to mail them to any address on receipt of price: Paper cover, $0.50; stiff bound, $0.75; elegant binding, $1.65.

Naturopathy embodies all natural healing methods, including Hydrotherapy (Priessnitz, Kneipp and Just's systems), Osteopathy, Heliotherapy (sun, light, and air cure), Hygienic and Physical and Mental Culture to the exclusion of all drugs and non-accidental surgery.

EDITORIAL DRIFT

by Benedict Lust

The Naturopath and Herald of Health, III(1), 32-33. (1902)

Naturopathy is a hybrid word. It is purposely so. No single tongue could distinguish a system whose origin, scope and purpose is universal—broad as the world, deep as love, high as heaven. Naturopathy was not born of a sudden or a happen-so. Its progenitors have for eons been projecting thoughts and ideas and ideals whose culminations are crystalized in the new Therapy. Connaro, doling out his few fixed ounces of food and drink each day in his determined exemplification of Dietotherapy; Priessnitz, agonizing despised and dejected through the long years of Hydropathy's travail; the Woerishofen priest, laboring lovingly in his little parish home for the thousands who journeyed Germany over for the Kneipp cure; Kuhne, living vicariously and dying a martyr for the sake of Serotherapy; A. T. Still, studying and struggling and enduring for his faith in Osteopathy; Bernarr Macfadden, fired by the will to make Physical Culture popular; Helen Willmans, threading the mazes of Mental Science, and finally emerging triumphant; Orrison Sweet Marden, throbbing in sympathy with human faults and failures, and longing to realize success to all mankind—these and hosts of others have brought into being single systems whose focal features are perpetuated in Naturopathy.

Jesus Christ—I say it reverently—knew the possibility of physical immortality. He believed in bodily beauty; He founded Mental Healing; He perfected Spirit-power. And Naturopathy will include ultimately the supreme forces that made the Man of Galilee omnipotent.

The scope of Naturopathy is from the first kiss of the new-found lovers to the burying of the centenarian whose birth was the symbol of their perfected oneness. It includes ideally every life-phase of the id, the embryo, the fetus, the birth, the babe, the child, the youth, the man, the lover, the husband, the father, the patriarch, the soul.

We believe in strong, pure, beautiful bodies thrilling perpetually with the glorious power of radiating health. We want every man, woman and child in this great land to know and embody and feel the truths of right living that mean conscious mastery. We plead for the renouncing of poisons from the coffee, white flour, glucose, lard, and like venom of the American table to patent medicines, tobacco, liquor and the other inevitable recourse of perverted appetite. We long for the time when an eight-hour day may enable every worker to stop existing long enough to live; when the sprit of universal brotherhood shall animate business and society and the church; when every American may have a little cottage of his own, and a bit of ground where he may combine Aerotherapy, Heliotherapy, Geotherapy, Aristophagy and nature's other forces with home and peace and happiness and the things forbidden to flat-dwellers; when people may stop doing and thinking and being for others and be for themselves; when true love and divine marriage and pre-natal culture and controlled parenthood may fill this world with germ-gods instead of humanized animals.

In a word, Naturopathy stands for the reconciling, harmonizing and unifying of nature, humanity and God.

Fundamentally therapeutic because men need healing; elementally educational because men need teaching; ultimately inspirational because men need empowering, it encompasses the realm of human progress and destiny.

Perhaps a word of appreciation is due Mr. John H. Scheel, who first used the term "Naturopathic" in connection with his Sanitarium "Badekur," and who has courteously allowed us to share the name. It was chosen out of some 150 submitted, as most comprehensive and enduring. All our present plans are looking forward some five or ten or fifty years when Naturopathy shall be the greatest system in the world.

Actually the present development of Naturopathy is pitifully inadequate, and we shall from time to time present plans and ask suggestions for the surpassing achievement of our world-wide purpose. Dietetics, Physical Culture and Hydropathy are the measures upon which Naturopathy is to build; mental culture is the means, and soul-selfhood is the motive.

If the infinite immensity of plan, plea and purpose of this particular magazine and movement were told you, you would simply smile in your condescendingly superior way and straightway forget. Not having learned as yet what a brain and imagination and a will can do, you consider Naturopathy an ordinarily innocuous affair, with a lukewarm purpose back of it, and an ebbing future ahead of it. Such is the character of the average wishy-washy health movement and tumultuous wave of reform.

Your incredulous smile would not discomfit us—we do not importune your belief, or your help, or your money. Wherein we differ from the orthodox self-labeled reformer, who cries for sympathy and cringes for shekels.

We need money most persistently—a million dollars could be used to advantage in a single branch of the work already definitely planned and awaiting materialization; and we need co-operation in a hundred different ways. But these are not the things we expect or deem best.

Criticism, fair, full and unsparing is the one thing of value you can give this paper. Let me explain. Change is the keynote of this January issue—in form, title, and make-up. If it please you, your subscription and a word to your still-benighted friends is ample appreciation. But if you don't like it, say so. Tell us wherein the paper is inefficient or redundant or ill-advised, how it will more nearly fit into your personal needs, what we can do to make it the broadest, deepest, truest, most inspiring of the mighty host of printed powers. *The most salient letter of less than 300 words will be printed in full, and we shall ask to present the writer with a subscription-receipt for life.*

By to-morrow you will probably have forgotten this request; by the day after you will have dropped back into your old ways of criminal eating and foolish drinking and sagged standing and congested sitting and narrow thinking and deadly fearing—until the next progress paper of New Thought or Mental Science or Dietetics or Physical Culture prods you into momentary activity.

Between now and December we shall tell you just how to preserve the right attitude, physical and mental, without a single external aid; and how, every moment of every day, to tingle and pulsate and leap with the boundless ecstasy of manhood consciously nearing perfection.

1903

The Origin Of The Naturopathic Society

Benedict Lust

Advertisement for courses offered by the American School of Naturopathy.

THE ORIGIN OF THE NATUROPATHIC SOCIETY

FROM THE NOTEBOOK OF BENEDICT LUST

by Benedict Lust

The Naturopath and Herald of Health, IV(1 & 2), 36-37. (1903)

Some ten years ago, a conclave of portentously solemn old-school doctors informed a certain fearful youth that he must die of consumption. Neither he nor they had ever heard of "Naturopathy"—in fact the word was not yet coined. But that declaration was the preface to the Naturopathic Society of America.

The youth, instead of dying, proceeded to defy the fiat of the prognosticators, and betook himself to Woerishofen, Germany, the home of the Kneipp-Cure. His determination, plus Father Kneipp's skill both restored the consumptive and animated him with a life's enthusiasm for bearing the tidings to a suffering world.

He visited the other German Sanitaria, and found his horizon broadening to include other methods besides Kneipp's. He discovered indeed that the percentage of cures as other Nature-Cure establishments was even greater than that of Woerishofen. So he studied the systems of Kuhne, Griebel, Walser, Lahmann, Bilz, Just, and other Natural Physicians.

The Kneipp-Cure had no dietetics to speak of, nor did it give due place to air-sun baths, massage, electrotherapy, mechanotherapy, physical culture, and suggestive therapeutics.

So the young apostle of Naturism had plans in view much broader and farther-reaching than the scope of the Kneipp headquarters, established in 1896. There was opposition from the very start. A prominent Kneipp practitioner already operating in the City announced positively:—"If you are exclusively Kneipp, I will cooperate with you; if not, I will work against you most zealously. And I shall see to it that all the Kneippianer already here become your foes."

This blind, narrow prejudice has held sway from the first. Many an old German customer still comes into the store for a Kneipp herb, refusing even to listen to the mention of Bilz or Just—just because they're not Kneipp. And so factions were awaiting the Kneipp-Verein, even before its organization in 1896. A few well-meaning fools started the craze of walking barefoot in Central Park—and all the Kneippists were blamed of course. Jealousies, spites and bickering soon came into evidence, chiefly between the original Kneipp devotees and the more liberal exponents of all Nature-Cure. Ignorant and immoral Kneipp-doctors somehow crept into the Verein; cliques sprang into being; general and unselfish interest abated; the lectures no longer awakened enthusiasm; the meetings began to lapse; and finally in the winter of 1901 the Society languished its last lisp. Its ashes and other burial paraphernalia are interred in a sequestered drawer of the Naturopathic Institute.

We have found it a thankless task to preach unity to Americanized Germans. There is a German saying: "Einigkeit macht stark." But they don't practice it, even where they proclaim the proverb. North and South Germans were never known to agree on anything, and when you export them to a cosmopolitan country like America, the situation gets more complex. Moreover the inherent principles of Naturopathy forbid the steins and pretzels that a German makes synonymous with congeniality.

We couldn't hold the Kneipp-Verein in Concert Halls, or behind the Family Entrance of a corner moonshine-factory. Beer and smoking were not allowed, and hence the society soon dwindled to a chatterfest of garrulous old women and self-advertising cranks.

Sometimes the lecturers themselves were half drunk, having acquired a dizzy whiskey characteristic in addition to the sedative beer quality that distinguishes home-grown Germans.

We began to be ashamed to own the name of Kneipp, just as a true Physical Culturist blushes to be classed among the mob of Mail Course criers that teach gymnastics on the type-writer.

And when the first Naturopathic meeting occurred in September, 1902, we felt a vast sense of relief that the former retinue of hose-pliers and compress-wringers had given place to a better class of true Kneippianer Naturists.

We have adopted special precautions for keeping the undesirables out of this new Society. Only people of recognized character and vouched for by a competent Committee will be admitted to membership. All classes will be provided for, from peasant to prince, but only the Truth-seekers from each class will be welcomed.

The account of the first meeting, given elsewhere in this number, proves that the leading thinkers, physicians and reformers of Greater New York are actively in sympathy with the Naturopathic idea and ideal. And though we have not asked or wished them to side openly with any movement for advancing Humanity, it is reassuring to know how fast the world is being prepared for the co-relation of Naturism, Humanism, and Divinism.

We have found, from closer touch with all the various specialty-cures, methods, and beliefs, that the Naturopathic conception is too comprehensive for most intellects to grasp. Even the so-called Nature Cure and New Thought exemplifiers are able to see but one side of the polygon. And that is why we specially need those of you who are both intelligent and sympathetic, in propagating Naturopathic principles. We want the little fraction of Truth that each specialist has worked out, without the dusty chalk-marks he makes in rectifying his computation. And we must be free to erase when and where and how we please, whether we rub out part of your little "sums" or not.

Read the stenographic report of the first Millenial Meeting. Then see if you don't understand better how all-inclusive Naturopathy aims to be.

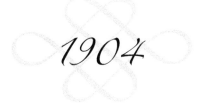

1904

Why We Oppose Vivisection
J. M. Greene

Father Kneipp And His Methods
Benedict Lust

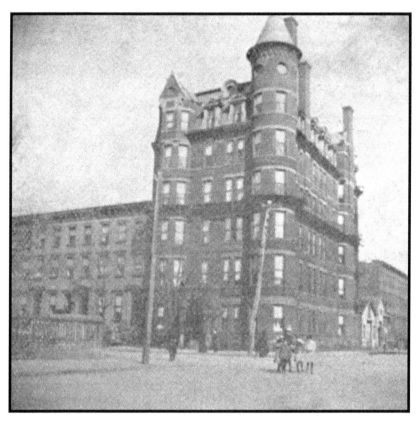

The New York Kneippianum, Madison Ave, Cor. 124th Street.

Why We Oppose Vivisection

By J. M. Greene

The Naturopath and Herald of Health, V(6), 121-125. (1904)

"There is no condition of experimentation possible with the influence of anesthesia, from which just conclusions can be formed! The thing is ridiculous. It is a reductio ab absurdum. Your "patient" must be either conscious or unconscious; if it is unconscious the experiment is admittedly "worthless;" if it is conscious its nervous system is so stimulated, and it is so upset by the torture, that no truth can be arrived at."

(Extracts from the last public utterance, April 20, 1899, of the late Prof. Lawson Tait, England's greatest abdominal surgery surgeon.)

Why do a large aggregate number of the thinking people of civilized countries opposed today the practice—called vivisection—of experimenting in medical laboratories on the bodies of living animals? This question is being constantly propounded in various forms, from that of sincere inquiry to one evidently containing a species of reproof. To propose to answer this question as concisely as possible, wasting no time over technical details, but presenting the subject as it would appeal everywhere to the intelligent and conscientious mind.

At the outset we may say that the practice of vivisection is opposed for two general reasons: because it violates both principles of common intelligence supposed to be at the foundation of all "science," and the moral law as well, which has ever decreed that the greater principle should never be sacrificed for the less—that those qualities which alone make this world a habitable one for human beings must not be offered up, a sacrifice to temporal advantage. As to the scientific aspect, one phase is well in concisely expressed in the quotation from Professor Tait at the head of this article. The abnormal condition caused either by severe pain or by anesthesia, as all can testify who have experienced either one, is an unknown and ever varying quantity, disarranging the bodily functions and throwing out of gear, as it were, the delicate parts of the living machine. Experimentation under such conditions is as if an expert astronomer, with all the perfected instruments of his profession, should endeavor to solve some intricate problem of the skies from the deck of a rocking boat! In this fact is found one great cause for the endless contradictions of all vivisectors—both self-contradictions and contradictions of each other—which have resulted in the immeasurable waste of animal life and suffering.

Another scientific error which alone would cost distrust in the unbiased mind, is the ignoring, in vivisection, of the numerous and vast differences existing between the various species. Vivisectors, such as Prof. Rutherford of England, have in candid moments acknowledged that whatever is "discovered" of value to man through animal experimentation must afterword be "tried on the man" himself before the "discovery" can benefit the human race! And in the vast majority of cases it is found that this "trying it on the man" afterward is a total failure. Even that great Sir Astley Cooper, through his mistake (caused by vivisection) of supposing that the process of repair in a bone broken inside the capsule was the same in human beings as in dogs, retarded surgical progress in that line for years, and made many cripples. The renowned surgeon, Sir Frederick Treves, of England, although denying that he is an anti-vivisectionist, yet has admitted in the British Medical Journal for November 5, 1898, that his experience on the intestines of dogs has so "harassed" him that he had "everything to unlearn!" These differences between the various species are nowhere more glaring than in the matter of drugs and medicines. Some small animals, the pigeon and the rabbit for instance, can take without injurious affect an amount of opium that would at once kill a human being; belladonna, so deadly to man, can be eaten by herbivorous animals with immunity; and like examples could be cited without number. Defenders of vivisection would have the lay public believe that drugs are always first tested on animals for the purpose of discovering their properties. Not so; the vast majority of drug tests are on human beings (with their consent), as can be ascertained by consulting such standard works of Clarke's "Materia Medica." And this has been found to be the only reliable method

Moreover, the unscientific nature of vivisection has been emphatically declared by impartial and disinterested scientific man of the highest standard—such as Sir Chas. Bell, Prof. Lawson Tait, Stephen Townsend, F. R. C. S., Deputy Surgeon General J. H. Thornton, Sir William Ferguson, F. R. S., Dr. Chas. Bell Taylor, F. F. C. S., and in this country by any physicians represented by such earnest investigators as the late Prof. James E. Garretson, Dr. William R. D. Blackwood and Dr. Matthew Woods, of Philadelphia. Public judgment is, however, blinded by the glamor thrown around this practice by active, influential and brainy men, selfishly interested in its promotion. These carry with them the majority of the medical profession, who, like the rest of human nature, float with the tide, very few of whom have ever seen a vivisection, and not 1% of whom ever performed one.

Now, as regards to the practical results of vivisection. Much enlightenment in this direction may be found in the fact that the great University of Harvard, although asked many times of late at the Massachusetts State House hearings on vivisection, to cite a single valuable discovery as a result of vivisection in their laboratories for the past 50 years, has been unable to do so! The very diseases for the cure of which vivisectors have been especially experimenting for the past 25 years, have meanwhile enormously increased in mortality; this includes diphtheria, cancer, pneumonia, cholera, Bright's disease, etc. This may be easily ascertained by consulting the reports of the Registrar-General for England. The most sweeping claims, regarding famous discoveries in the past, are constantly made, but on examination they prove unwarranted. Sir Chas. Bell himself disclaimed that his discovery of the functions on the anterior and posterior nerves with the results of vivisection. Hunter's operations for aneurism of the artery, so often cited, was first tried and proved on human beings; animals never have this disease. Anesthetics were discovered through experiments by medical men, Morton and Simpson, on themselves; and Harvey's additional facts regarding the circulation of the blood, largely gathered through observation of the valves in the veins of a dead body, could at any time have been demonstrated, as stated by Prof. Tait, with a dead body and an injecting syringe. "Pasteurism" has not diminished the mortality from "hydrophobia," but has caused many deaths from laboratory poisoning with the virus of that disease; it is denounced by such authorities as Prof. Lutaud, Dr. Dolan, Dr. Dulles, Prof. Spitzka, and the late renowned Prof. Peter. The modern serums have utterly failed; as the L.L.D. of England declared August 2, 1899 before the British Medical Association, they "cannot be proved to have saved a single human life or lessened in any appreciable degree the load of human misery." Their most famous example, "diphtheria antitoxin," boomed, as it has been, with the most consummate commercial ability, has yet been followed by an increased mortality from that disease in many parts of the world. The vital question, moreover, is not "Has anything of value been discovered through vivisection?" but, "Has anything been discovered that could have been discovered in no other way?" From time immemorial the most important facts, useful in the treatment of disease, have been gained through observation at the bedside, combined with anatomical study and post mortem examination, and in later times, through work with the microscope. But these invaluable and proven means of research have of late years been to a great extent neglected for the new and fascinating method of vivisection, to the discredit of the profession and the increase of disease. The laws of hygiene, as well, have been grossly slighted, and in place of Nature's beneficent great extent neglected for the new and cleanliness, air, diet and physical and mental development, we have offered to us the loathsome products that disease propagated in the bodies of tortured animals, and are told to inject these abominations into the life current of ourselves and our children!

When, however, we come to the ethical aspect of the question, the real inwardness of this practice is revealed. In the first place, the fact is undeniable that great cruelties are constantly perpetrated. The vivisectors themselves, when in a confidential mood, acknowledge this, and the physiological magazines are full of details appalling to the humane reader. "Anesthetics"—so constantly used in extenuation and when the public conscience is to be calmed—are here to a great extent a delusion. Many experiments, such as those on the nervous system, the vital organs, circulation, etc., and those with drugs, would be utterly "vitiated" by the use of anesthetics; while experiments involving lingering and painful disease (often referred to by the vivisector as "involving the mere prick of a pin") they are of course, absent. In descriptions of experiments the drugs morphia and chloral are sometimes mentioned as if they are anesthetics. These drugs are, however, not true anesthetics, but simply narcotics, producing at times a stupor, but not destroying pain. Indeed, under certain circumstances, morphia, on dogs for example, acts as a violent stimulant instead! Moreover, in place of anesthetics, it is common for vivisectors to use a drug called curare, which paralyzes the nerves of motion, but in no way acts as a deadener of pain. When this awful poison is employed the animal can be kept alive only by artificial respiration—in other words, air is continually pumped in and out of the lungs by means of an engine.

The practice of vivisection is also one of wide extent, notwithstanding the habit of referring to its victims as "a few" rabbits, or "a few" guinea pigs. The most sensitively organized creatures are sacrificed in great numbers. It is a regular occupation, carried on by teachers for the purpose of demonstrating well known facts, by students for the "practice" they may acquire and by great numbers of physiologists throughout the world. Animals are vivisected by thousands in single establishments, in many of which, such as the Paris Academy of medicine, they are bred for that purpose alone. Pasteur in his experiments with rabies sacrificed so many dogs that, as he wrote, the number had "passed beyond the possibility of numbering them." Taking this into consideration, its nature and extent, the amount of suffering caused by this practice may, to certain degree, be realized.

It is at this point that the question comes before the honest and thinking mind, and will not be put aside—What right has man, in the name of honor and conscience, to perpetuate these cruelties? What right has he, being the stronger, to make a curse to them of the poor lives of the creatures about him—to crush them beneath the heel of his egotism and tear them with the engines of his cupidity and ambition? This question has never been answered by either the vivisector or his apologists, from the callow medical student with a taste for research to the dignified Bishop who brings, or seeks to bring, the influence of his church in defense of his old time friends of some vivisecting University. It has never been answered because it never can be. The vivisectionist can ever invent some new "scientific" claim, as the old are one by one proved false, but from the moral standpoint he is without defense. The most he can do, when brought face-to-face with the moral law, is to employ the familiar *tu quoque* argument and cite other shameless cruelties to the animal world, as if these, as a matter of course, were justifiable. But, to be brief, *who says so?* Who says we have the right to seize upon the beautiful horse, the patient cattle, the gentle sheep, the faithful dog and all the breathing works of Nature, and desecrate them on the altar of our appetites, our greed or our curiosity? *Who says so?* Give me no answer with the odor upon it of some foul and cruel superstition, always the bulwark of tyranny and wrong, but a clean and honest answer born of justice and common sense. Tell me why the small and weak are not entitled to their happiness as well as the great and strong—why, in obedience to anything but an all-absorbing egotism, we, the self-appointed arbiters of "justice," are forever violating the first principles of justice. But the only answer is silence. The driveling query, whether one would "sacrifice the child for the rabbit or the rabbit for the child," is not even an attempt at an answer—it has its source only in the vacuum of the sophistry hopelessly impotent, for no one has ever dreamed of sacrificing the child for the rabbit. The domain of justice cannot be bound by the limits of one race or species. The vicious idea that the means is sanctified by the end has been the excuse for every atrocity. The fallacy that undeserved suffering is less undeserved because endured by the helpless is the flimsiest in the domain of logic; and the same excuses that are given for the vivisection of animals would apply even more strongly to the vivisection of the pauper, the idiot and the outcast. No one perceives this more clearly than does the vivisectionist; hence his studied evasion of the questions outlined above. Would that serious thought might be given to those questions also by certain opponents of vivisection who now by their daily life invite the irreverent flings of the vivisector.

But the moral evils of vivisection are not confined to the act of injustice inflicted upon the animal. Nature is not safely abused, and the human soul, calloused by cruelty to its humbler associates, will become a curse to its own kind. By the encouragement of this practice upon those who have no power to resist and no voice to protest, we have slowly but surely awakened the demon of human vivisection whose shadow is already dark over the medical world. Men, women and children have been, and are, through inoculation, drug poisoning and unnecessary operations, being vivisected secretly, and sometimes not so secretly, in the hospitals of the poor—and the end is not in sight. The hunger for "physiological research" is simply sharpened by its unavailing attempts upon the "lower" species and longs for more appropriate material. This deadly menace has already become a powerful factor in keeping away from the free hospitals many unfortunates who realize their greater danger, in the presence of an unseen foe.

A great danger to society is also present in the fact that the moral callousness generated by the practice is liable to extend widely among the general public (as to some extent it already has) through familiarity with the statements and claims of vivisectors.

Why, then, in brief, do we oppose the practice of vivisection? We oppose it because it, itself, is opposed to both humanity and science. Because what is wrong with Nature under such conditions is valueless, as it was from the tortured prisoner of old. Because, although some facts may have been thus blundered upon amid the mass of delusions and contradictions, yet by it the scientific mind has been diverted from rational and humane channels which would have produced results a hundred fold greater. Because, in comparison to the terrible cost of this method—cost in time, energy, moral retrogression and the suffering of sensitive creatures—all the "beneficial results" have been but a "drop in the bucket." Because it is wrong to do evil that good may come. Because Justice allows no boundary line of species, and the right of the weak to exemption from pain is as sacred as the right of the strong. In short, because it is full-time that the "right of might," so long the gospel of savagery, should cease to be that of a civilized people.

FATHER KNEIPP AND HIS METHODS

by Benedict Lust

Naturopath and Herald of Health, V(7), 145-149. (1904)

[Being the substance of an address delivered on April 14th, 1904, at the Cosmological Center, 36 W. 27th St., New York City.]

A number of years ago, a young man then twenty–two years of age, went back to Germany to die of consumption—"given up" by all the medical men who had anything to do with him. He had tried homeopathy and allopathy, and other methods, but without result.

The young man went to Woerishoefen in Bavaria, and saw Father Kneipp; the good Father looked him over, heard all he had to say, and at the conclusion of the interview said, "I don't know whether I can put you together again or not, but I will see what we can do."

The young man started to take the cure, and his health began to improve from the very start. In eight months he was in the enjoyment of perfect health.

When he proved in his own experience the value of Father Kneipp's treatment for himself, he determined to devote his life to transmitting to others the benefits of the system of healing that had done so much for him.

He set to work to study that system, and told Father Kneipp that he should go back to America and teach the people there how to cure disease by means of it. The Father slapped him on the back heartily and said, "Follow the system in America!"

That young man was myself. I can truly say that I have faithfully filled my promise to the very utmost of my ability.

Incidentally, it may be said that Mr. Lust is a tall, well-built, vigorous man, with bright eyes, clear complexion and every outward evidence of superabundant good health, high animal spirits, and physical vigor. Nobody, to look at him, would have the least idea that he had ever had a day's sickness in his life—much less that he had ever been as sick as he described in his address. As a living advertisement of the virtues of the Kneipp system of healing it would be very hard to improve upon Mr. Lust himself.—Reporter.)

Father Kneipp was a man of very simple life, but he possessed a large share of personal magnetism that created confidence and love and made people willing to obey him promptly unquestioningly. As can be seen by his portraits, his face was full of character. It was distinguished by the size of his nose, and the distance between the nose and the lips.

He was a tall man with a sturdy, robust figure and his manner of speaking sounded rather rough in the ears of city people.

He was born and brought up in the country, and had but few educational advantages. He early desired to be a priest, but he only realized that wish by hard work and by enlisting the sympathy of a priest, who gave him valuable aid.

He worked so hard at his studies that his health gave way after three years of high-school and he was sent home to die, the doctors telling him they had no hope of his recovery.

At this time a book fell into his hands that had been written on the Priessnitz Water Cure—the father of hydro-therapy—or healing by means of water.

Father Kneipp did not originate water-curing, but he modernized and improved the practice found already in existence. Fifteen years ago people were much stronger than they are now, and could stand much more vigorous treatment. Kneipp, in those days, practiced what was called the "horse cure"—so called because of the strength of constitution needed to stand the applications. He himself broke the ice in the Danube for four weeks to give himself the treatment prescribed by Priessnitz, and feeling none the worse at the end of that time—though no marked improvement was manifest—he returned to the college to resume his studies. There he earned the title of the "water doctor," and practiced his methods on the other students, mostly at the fountain in the courtyard and late at night, after the professors had gone to bed. There he effected two cures that were so successful that he made life-long friends of his grateful patients, who helped a great deal after he became a priest.

At first when he became a priest he devoted himself to the duties of his parish but he could not help trying to cure the people whom he found to be sick. Several times these efforts conflicted with his official duties as a priest, and once he even found himself under arrest.

In Munich a judge said to him, "You are trying to make criminals, nobody needs the water-cure." Father Kneipp replied, "You need it for yourself; for I can see that you will be a dead man in six months."

And the event proved that Father Kneipp's words were true.

In another court the judge asked him: "Can you cure rheumatism? Yes, I can!"

The next day he came to the establishment to take the cure.

The success of the treatment soon made it popular and such heavy demands were made upon him that the Bishop forbade his doing any more of this work. He did his best to obey for a time until an incident happened that decided all his future life.

One night he was sent for to treat a woman said to be dying; he sent back word that he could not come. Again the summons came, and again he refused. About eleven o'clock he went to bed, but found himself unable to sleep for thinking of the woman, and of the possibility of her dying because he refused to go to her assistance. At last he got up, saying, "I'm going to see the woman, and stick to the work of curing the sick from this time on."

That night settled the question of his practicing, and his success soon proved that God had called him to heal the sick by his methods. In 1886 he published his book *My Water Cure* in German, so that the readers could cure themselves at home without coming to him. But instead of lessening the number of people visiting him for advice, it greatly increased them. Woerishofen was filled with strangers from all parts of Europe. Hotels were built, and the out-of-the-way village became a town of 24,000 inhabitants.

The agents used in Kneipp's healing methods are air, light, sunshine, and diet, as well as water. But, primarily, the Kneipp methods are intended to prevent sickness by keeping well people in good health, to cause robust persons to live plain, simple lives, and to harden the

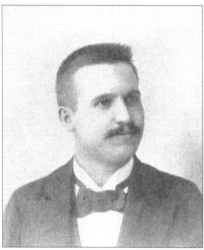 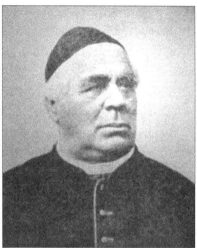

Benedict Lust.   Fr. Sebastien Kneipp.

constitution by means of the natural agents just named—not by means of drugs and medicines. Father Kneipp's book gives full directions for both, the preservation of health and the cure of sickness. The book has been translated into fifty-two languages, and in the German language alone 136 editions have been issued.

To an average normally healthy man Kneipp would say: "Keep your constitution hardened and robust, and protected against the weather, so that you do not become sensitive to cold." But he prescribed washings and ablutions, and not sponge baths as people usually take them.

A beginner should just take cold water out of a basin and apply it quickly to the arms, chest and upper part of the body, and then put on the clothing at once—without drying the skin with a towel.

Next day the other parts of the body should be treated in the same way, but no towel must be used before putting on the clothes again.

The body must always be kept warm and exercise must be taken at once so as to promote and sustain quick reaction of the skin.

After a while a half-bath may be taken. Get into a bathtub full of cold water, sit in it while you count "4," get out quickly, and dress immediately, without using towel.

The use of the towel causes the body to lose warmth. Water left on the skin retains warmth as it is evaporated by the heat of the body. Coarse underwear should be worn, as fine garments stick the body and prevent the air from having free access to the skin; therefore the material should be of coarse linen or cotton.

This half bath may be taken about three times a week.

No item of treatment should be continued long enough for the system to "get used" to it; because then it will fail to produce good effects. Therefore it is wise to change the order of different details of treatment taken, or omitting some for a while and then taking again. This principle holds good in all applications of the water cure.

A full bath is like a half bath, except that all the body is submerged.

Among other applications that can be used at home are douches. These are not shower baths (in which water comes down from above or around the patient), but can be given by water cannon or a hose with, say, 1 ½ inch opening. The water just runs over the skin, but is not directed against the body with any force.

The first of these is the knee-douche. This is very useful for drawing the blood from the head and strengthening nervous patients; also to induce sleep in case of insomnia.

The application begins at the heel, and goes upward at the back of the leg to the knee. The water is applied until the skin get red; it is stopped then, in order to avoid the loss of heat and vitality.

Then there are hip douches; back douches (very useful for strengthening the back and spinal cord), chest douches, and douches for various other parts of the body, the mode being the same in all cases, and no towel being used before clothing is resumed.

The lightning gush is like the douche, except that force is applied to the water, the attendant holding the hose about six feet from the patient.

Cold water applications always produce heat and increase vitality and the different douches cause better metabolism, or assimilation of food; therefore patients need more food, more rest and more exercise while taking them. People who are working every day should not take more than two or three a week.

Kneipp did not oppose all steam baths; properly applied they will relieve cold in the head and the chest or the limbs; but he put herbs in the water of the vapor baths and thereby made them more effective. Every warm application of the kind should, however, be followed by cold douche or other method of treatment.

Packs. The principle is a wet sheet wound round the body from the arms to the knees, the water used being cold for a strong patient, but warm for weak one. It should be kept on for half or three quarters of an hour. It is very useful for dissolving impurities of the system, and causing it to excrete morbid matter. It should always be applied with care.

The Spanish Mantle covers the body, the patient being wrapped in a sheet and put to bed. It produces a good sweat, and the patient should be washed down with cold water afterwards.

For sore throat, neck bandages wet with cold water, may be used; they must be renewed every ten minutes. The bandages must never be allowed to remain on after they get warm, and no air must be permitted to get between the skin and bandage.

A good way to cure colds is by a half-bath, taken three or four times a day, with cold water alone. The trouble is not really with the nose or the throat in itself, but exists all over the body, although it may be more manifest in these special organs. The impurities in the system are unable to escape by the pores of the skin, and therefore try to get out in the form of phlegm, etc., through the membranes. Vapor baths are good, and so are packs, but the half-bath previously described, is the simplest method.

Diet. Kneipp was not a vegetarian or a fruitarian, but his system is a kind of bridge from the old system of diet to these new ones. He never told anyone to give up anything all at once. If a man were in the habit of drinking fifteen glasses of beer a day, he would reduce the number to seven; if ten cigars were smoked a day, he would make it five; three meat meals a day would be cut down to one. To people used to taking much medicine he would give herb teas of various kinds.

One of his principles was to get city people out of the city into the country; and he had a marvelous capacity for handling people, and managing them so as to make them do what he wanted them.

He was one of the busiest men in the whole German Empire, and often had 4000 people to hear him when he lectured. I had four interviews with him altogether—one of them at five o'clock in the morning.

He stood up for mixed diet of meat and vegetables; he ate meat himself but recognized that vegetariansim was good, if the dietary were properly arranged.

Father Kneipp drank two or three glasses of beer in a year, but he was not a crank on the subject of intoxicants.

He was against the use of white flour, declaring that the best part of the wheat was removed in the milling. He believed in soups made of cereals with vegetable or milk stock, but not in soups made from meat; also in plenty of sauerkraut.

Father Kneipp died at the age of 76 from overwork; he usually worked from 4 A.M. till 11 P.M. every day in the week. For the last few years of his life he certainly did not take proper care of himself. Still it must be borne in mind that he had been "given up by the doctors" at the age of 28.

As a priest he possessed private means, that he was not obliged to treat people for money, and he did not care for money at all, in itself. One of the Rothschild's offered him 50,000 Florins if he would go to Vienna to treat him, and he refused to go, not even answering the letter. He traveled in Germany and Italy and went to Paris once, where he effected some marvelous cures. In one year he cured the Archduke Joseph of Austria of a kidney disease of thirty-six years' standing. As a token of his gratitude the Archduke gave 150,000 Florins for a public park in Woerishofen.

Father Kneipp established six institutions of healing and philanthropy. He built the children's asylum in 1892, where 3,000 "incurable" cases have been treated by nature methods. Then another building for old men and old women, to which only the poor are admitted.

There institutions at a distance from the city for certain diseases such as cancer.

The Father was very democratic in all his ways. Each person who visited him received a number as he entered the waiting apartment, and no rank or social position would procure any advancement over the poorest person who had previously arrived.

A certain princess staying at a hotel had sent four or five messages by servants for him to visit her, but without result. She then sent a lady-in-waiting, who told the father that she held this position in the princess's household. Instead of being impressed with the dignity of the messenger, however, he said: "Oh, I call that a servant-girl; when I am through with all these other people, I will come, and not before!"

An Austrian prince, on leaving Woerishofen, after a successful course of treatment, called on the Father as he left the town and handed him a purse of gold for a present. He took it and put it in his deep pocket. A little while after a poor Romanian woman came to ask him to give her the money to get home again to Bucharest, being needed. He dived down into his pocket and handed her the purse that he had just received from the Archduke, which contained 800 Marks.

Since Father Kneipp took up the Nature cure, about 250 health movements along similar lines have been started, some of which have done much good. None, however, was as good as his, which has been taken up by even the medical world in Europe. And in all parts of America are to be found institutions in which Kneipp's system of healing is worked out in greater or less detail.

> *To an average normally healthy man Kniepp would say: "Keep your constitution hardened and robust, and protected against the weather, so that you do not become sensitive to cold."*

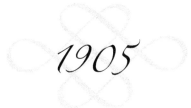

1905

WHO ARE THE QUACKS?
FROM THE OPTHAMOLOGIST

———

THE MEDICAL "FAKIR"
A. JUSTICE SEEKER, S.A.B.

———

OUR MEDICAL LAWS
BENEDICT LUST

THE MEDICAL QUESTION

The Truth About Official Medicine and Why We Must Have Medical Freedom

Medical Laws vs. Human Rights and Constitution. The Great Need of the Hour. What Constitutes the True Science and Art of Healing

By A. A. ERZ, N. D., D. C.

HERE is a book that cheers one like a draught of ozone after having breathed the mephitic vapors of the philosophy of official medicine, that exploits the immorality of vivisection, and swears by the unscientific and useless products of the torture trough.

It consists of 600 pages, written by the trenchant pen of one who is master of his subject. It embodies the revolt of the latest and most efficient school of medical healing against the tyranny and ignorance of the drug doctors, who, while attacking symptoms, fail to understand the need of the higher practice of treating the causes of disease instead. The charlatanry and inefficiency of official medicine has reason to be envious of the successes of the natural school whose philosophic practices are here fully manifested.

Dr. Erz makes very clear his position in the art of healing. He is an enthusiastic Naturopath. He believes that when a man becomes ill, he should employ the natural forces of hydropathy, diet, exercise, sunshine, electricity, mechano-therapy, massage, and all the healing agencies that have proven their worth as prophylactics, and their ability to arouse the inherent restorative power for health that resides in every organism. His information is illuminating in the highest degree.

He is the sworn enemy of the "scientific medicine" of the allopaths, that consists of poisonous drugs on the one hand, and the equally poisonous and wholly dangerous serums, inoculations and vaccines on the other, that form a body of medical superstition that is propagating disease rather than curing it. He discusses, one by one, the most loudly-praised products of medical research, and proves them either to be utterly useless, or of deadly danger to the duped and unsuspecting patient.

In support of his statements, he quotes the opinions of the greatest exponents of official medicine who confess that allopathic medicine has produced more misery and premature death than famine, pestilence and war combined. As Billroth says, "Our progress is over mountains of corpses."

He proves that the American Medical Association, and the various State and County Associations affiliated therewith, form one vast engine of oppression, armed with legal power to harass, crush, and if possible destroy, the true saviors of mankind, the exponents of natural healing, whose activities naturally discredit official medicine. By legally securing a monopoly of practising medicine, THEY ARE ABLE TO MAKE IT MORE OF A CRIME TO CURE A PERSON THAN TO KILL HIM.

He shows how easy it is to understand why the unthinking legislator favors official medicine to the exclusion of the natural school of therapy. The psychological pressure of an institution, no matter how despotic its use of power may be, or how false and deadly its products are, that has its roots deeply rooted in history, is vastly greater on the unenlightened mind, than a true and noble institution that was born but yesterday—where man does not know conservatism rules.

Dr. Erz fully proves that the so-called remedies of medical research are violations of every law of nature, of health, of life, and a disregard of every principle of physiology, biology and therapeutics.

The people were never consulted about these laws, and never asked for them

They are the product of medical feudalism, which means intolerance, injustice and brutality, instead of charity, justice and dignity. The people should rise in their might and stay the infamous activities of these medical malefactors.

It is a startling indictment of humanity that its saviors are never recognized until the advance guard, and many of the main army, are killed, or trodden underfoot, and official medicine in America, the glorious Land of Freedom, is busy at this moment, as it has been for many years past, in hunting down the drugless practitioner, whose only fault is the fact that he cures patients by natural methods, where the vendors of rotten pus have signally failed. He is arrested, and heavily fined, or thrown into jail for the offense of practising medicine without a pus-vendor's license.

Dr. Erz rightly advocates the urgent need of a great Academy of Natural Healing to convince the thinking masses of the superiority of the Natural Healing System, and to protect it against all misrepresentations and abuses, and assure its efficiency and permanent success. Medical Freedom is the great need of the hour to prove that Nature's constructive laws overshadow all ignorance, superstition and ambition. As the exponent of a standard of drugless healing, and as a monitor, mentor, and defence of humanity from rapacity and superstition, such an institution would be of enormous value to mankind.

Dr. Erz's work is a standard contribution to the great propaganda of Drugless Therapy that is sweeping over the land. No drugless practitioner can afford to be without its inspiring companionship. It marks an epoch in the history of the grand science and art of Natural Healing.

Price, in cloth, postpaid, $5.00; paper cover, $4.00.

THE NATURE CURE PUBLISHING CO., BUTLER, N. J.

Medical Laws vs. Human Rights and Constitution, a book by A. A. Erz, N.D., D.C.

WHO ARE THE QUACKS?

from **The Ophthalmologist**

The Naturopath and Herald of Health, VI(3), 61-65. (1905)

The code of ethics of the American Medical Associations has never before been printed—probably because no member would have the cheek to stand for it. Here it is in cold type; let every reader compare it with the conduct of the trust doctors of his acquaintance and see if it is not unadulterated truth.

1. We were first in the field, hence we are the only "regulars."

2. We will have no professional intercourse with graduates of other schools, under any circumstances, nor with graduates of colleges of our own school not recognized by our executive committee.

3. No college shall be recognized by our committee unless its management tacitly, at least, recognizes the authority of the committee by conforming to certain rules prescribed by it for the government of our medical colleges.

4. Any member of our association who advertises in the newspapers shall be expelled—provided that a simple card announcing his name and location or any free notices he may receive in the press shall not be considered advertising.

5. The fact that we are conspicuous members of society affords opportunity for newspaper interviews, which, of course, give the doctor prominence but it shall be considered a violation of this code for any young doctor to have himself interviewed—that is a privilege to which only the more mature leaders are entitled. Of course we can not punish the young doctor who does this, but we will discourage such forwardness on the part of the younger generation and will use our influence with the newspapers to suppress such unseemly outbreaks.

6.   We pledge ourselves to never let an opportunity pass to speak disrespectfully, even sneeringly of other creeds, because our silence would be giving our consent to their existence. The founders of those creeds were revolutionists, rebels, who denied the authority of our committees.

7.   Of course, some of them have become so powerful that our medical practice acts were about to be overthrown by the courts and we were compelled to recognize them in a legal sense, but no member should forget that national and state laws are one thing and our laws are another.

8.   We have, thus far, been able to control the public medical service so far as the nation is concerned, but in states and municipalities the other sects have secured a foothold. This must be discouraged at all hazards, and to that end every member must make it as unpleasant as possible for the health officer who does not recognize our authority.

9.   We, being the only orthodox school of medicine, and having the greatest influence with the public, must use it judiciously to prevent the exploitation of advanced ideas until we have investigated them and if they be good we will claim them as ours and denounce the claims of the others as fraudulent and impudent.

10. In order to protect the public we must be ever ready to denounce as frauds and insane quacks any and all who through books and periodicals, controlled by them, proclaim that our methods are mistaken in any particular. Of course we have modified our practices as we have gained knowledge from experience, but until we have information through regular channels it shall be violation of this code for any member to adopt new ideas.

11. Caution. There is a strong sentiment abroad that because we have failed to prove that medicine is a science, we have no rights to the protection afforded us by practice acts, and as such sentiments are openly expressed by a

wealthy and powerful faction among laymen, therefore be diplomatic. Of course, as individuals, we can ridicule faith-healing and drugless systems of all kinds, but it is advisable, in reconstructing our medical laws, to cater to the mental methods because they have a large following so far as minor ills go and we cannot afford to offend Christian prejudices or we will lose the support of the churches.

12. Every member should make it a point to enlist the ministry in our behalf, hence half rates or free services should be granted them, and they should be impressed with the immense value of our services so they will proclaim our worth from their pulpits. It is advisable to join some church.

13. Certain people, who are otherwise good citizens have taken up mechanical methods of ascertaining causes of human ills and in a few months learned how to relieve many of what we have believed to be incurable chronic ills. They call themselves Neurologists, Ophthalmologists, Hydropaths, N.Ds, Naturopaths, Hygienists, Osteopaths, etc. These are the most dangerous classes that have arisen and must be suppressed, but in doing this public sentiment must be first arrayed against them, hence if one of them has any social or political or financial standing let him alone, until we shall have suppressed those of his class who are not so fortunately situated; then we can go after the strongest.

14. Judges of the courts are good men to have on our side. They are learned men and we must approach them with the suggestion that these new sects cannot be worthy because they do not have four-year courses, and have no right to a standing in law. This will be a strong point with them, because it will impress them as being logical.

15. In dealing with the public be reticent. It is unethical to

converse with patients in language which will be comprehensive. If asked for an explanation of a case in simple language, say it cannot be given, that unless the patient has been educated in medicine it would be impossible for him or her to understand. If explanation is insisted upon exhibit indignation at the want of confidence implied give up the case. Dignity must be maintained.

16. In case of controversy over fees with dissatisfied patients it is better to compromise than go to law where there is always danger of unpleasant notoriety, and if subpoenaed as a witness in such a case, no matter if the defendant is irregular, let your evidence protect him if possible—you may need him in a similar capacity at any moment.

17. If you have a puzzling case where the family desire consultation, be firm in your demands for a physician of your own school, because the irregular schools do not practice as we do and if the consulting doctor changes treatment and the patient recovers it will be to your discredit and to the discredit of regular medicine. Dr. G.M. Gould truly says: "It is better that a patient die under regular treatment than that one recover by irregular methods."

18. Organize, attend your meetings, suppress jealousies among yourselves. Of course we have hundreds of unlearned, even ignorant regulars, but we were compelled to take them into our colleges without qualifications or they would have gone to irregular schools, and we must stand by them. If handled rightly they can be kept in line and they can often be relied upon to do things publicly that we want done but cannot do ourselves. Then, if we fail in our fight for supremacy we can use them as scape-goats.

19. Any medical journal that prints inquiries for advice shall be regarded as unethical because it will constantly expose the profession to suspicion by the laity into whose hand such journals chance to fall. They will consider the inquiries confessions of incompetency.

20.   No doctor shall be considered ethical who patents an invention or keeps secret any remedy which might be used with profit by the profession. Genius should seek no reward from the craft.

21.   When we, as an association, endorse a serum, it must be accepted as authoritative and anyone who has the temerity to ask for proofs must be either ignored, ridiculed, or suppressed; it shall be the duty of secretaries of state boards to utilize the funds collected for state licenses for this purpose.

22.   The big newspapers of the country get much of their revenue from the patient medicine fakir and advertising doctor, but they print our contributions as pure reading matter because we do not advertise individuals except in a complimentary way and on general principles, thus we have a powerful ally at little cost, and can save our money to secure favorable legislation.

23.   Inasmuch as we are unable to guarantee good results in any case with any reasonable assurance to ourselves and if we guarantee one and win, the public might want us to guarantee all cases, it shall be unethical to practice on that plan and anyone who does it shall be denounced as a quack.

24.   Members of our associations who take post-graduate courses at irregular schools shall be regarded as having forfeited the respect of regulars, because their act is an insinuation they are not satisfied with recognized authorities.

25.   The traditions of regular medicine are sacred and anyone who scouts our text-book authorities must be crazy, and shall be treated with silent contempt.

26.   Never miss an opportunity to refer to medicine as an honorable and philanthropic profession, laying stress on the free work we do; that will in a measure account for the notorious lack of financial responsibility among us.

27. The tendency among doctors of the present day is toward independence, seclusion, segregation and isolation, these are held to be faiths that should be overcome. We must hang together.

28. Contagious and infectious diseases after the preventive has been administered, it would arouse suspicion in the minds of the laity. Always leave a loop-hole.

29. It shall be the duty of members who are health officers of cities, towns, etc., to keep statistics in such a manner that they will support our claims. And when any one expresses doubt or wants to argue the questions of serums, statistics, etc., decline with dignity.

30. Those who charge that vaccination, antitoxin and other serums produce cancer, tuberculosis, erysipelas, rheumatism, etc., must be ignored if possible, and the public be given to understand such talk can only come from ignorant brains. Make them as ridiculous as possible.

31. Our Louisiana Association is the most progressive of all the states because it has secured the enactment of the following section in its medical practice act:

    Sec. 14. Be it further enacted, etc., that if any person shall practice medicine in any of its departments in this State, without first having obtained the certificate herein provided for, or contrary to the provisions of this act the Board of Medical Examiners created by this act may through their respective presidents cause to issue in any competent court a writ of injunction forbidding and enjoining said person from further practicing medicine in any of its departments in this State, until such person shall have first obtained the certificate herein provided for and under the provisions of this act.

    That said injunction shall not be subject to being released upon bond. That in the same suit in which said injunction may be applied for, the said boards through their respective presidents aforesaid, may sue for and demand of the defendant a penalty not to exceed one hundred dollars; and in addition thereto attorney's fees not to exceed fifty dollars, besides the costs of court; judgment for which penalty, attorney's fees, and costs may be rendered in the same judgment in which the injunction may be made absolute.

That the trial of said proceeding shall be summary, and be tried by the judge without the intervention of a jury.

32. Texas Association is the most derelict of all, in that its medical law contains the following paragraph:

Section 13. Any person who shall practice medicine, surgery or midwifery in this State in violation of the provisions of this act shall be fined not less than fifty dollars nor more than five hundred dollars for each offense or by both fine and imprisonment not exceeding six months and it shall not be lawful for him or her to recover by action, suit, motion, or warrant, any compensation for services which may be claimed to have been rendered by him or her as such physician, surgeon or midwife; provided, that the provisions of this act do not apply to persons treating disease who do not prescribe or give drugs or medicines.

It is announced, however, that an effort will be made this winter to have the offensive part of the paragraph, contained in the last two lines, stricken out, so that we will have a monopoly.

33. In the matter of transferring cases from one physician to another it is all right to divide the fees—unless the public catches on, when it shall be declared a breach of ethics. These matters are usually smoothed over, however, in the manner indicated by the following report, taken from the Chicago Tribune, November 19:

The introduction by Dr. E. C. Dudley at the meeting of an amendment to the constitution prohibiting its members from making any division of their fees with other surgeons was the signal for a discussion regarding the part taken by the president, Dr. J. Clarence Webster, and the secretary, Dr. Palmer Findley, in the recent exposure of the division fees.

Dr. Findlet suggested the scheme to a reporter of the Tribune, dictated the decoy letter, and selected the names of the surgeons to whom they were to be sent by checking them off in a medical directory. Dr. Webster was consulted frequently. He revised and made corrections in the letter. When the answers were sent on to Chicago, they were turned over to Dr. Findley by the reporter, and the reporter later secured them from Dr. Webster.

Dr. Webster and Dr. Findley made statements regarding their actions. The discussion which followed was participated in by several other of the physicians present, and is said to have been heated until toward the close of the meeting, which did not adjourn until midnight.

Later, speakers, it was said, strove to bring about harmony, and the spirit manifested toward the last indicated that much of the bitterness had been overcome and that for the best interests of the society and the profession it was decided to take a lenient view of the ethical offense which some of those present thought, their president and secretary had committed.

The decision is said to have been reached that the incident should be closed as far as that society is concerned.

Of course, the conduct of the two doctors was reprehensible, morally, because the exposure tended to discredit our honor, but what could we do? If we disciplined them they might kick over the traces and do even worse things, and it was therefore wisest to let them down easy and hope they will not sign in. Their act was probably prompted by jealousy—possibly superinduced by hunger.

34. Never miss an opportunity to boom vaccination and anti-toxin. For administering the former, there's from 25 cents to a dollar in each case, and for the latter there is from $3 to $5.

35. If any layman or irregular doctor asks why we wear whiskers and go with impunity from contagious and infectious diseases to other patients, declare we have a method of disinfection which renders us immune from either taking or carrying disease. And if no one asks why we do not use it on the public instead of isolating cases at homes or in hospitals, tell them our process only works on regular doctors. If they refuse to believe it, we will have the legislatures pass laws compelling them to recognize us as supernatural beings.

THE MEDICAL "FAKIR"

by A. Justice Seeker, S.A.B.

The Naturopath and Herald of Health. VI(3), 74-75. (1905)

A paper entitled "Medical Quacks, Their Methods and Dangers," was read before the Society of Jurisprudence by the honored counsel for the Medical Society of the County of New York.

In part the honorable gentleman said: "There are two big classes of quacks. First, those who have attended a medical school for a time and have failed in their examinations, or those who have practiced in other States and counties; second, those who have no medical education whatever.

"Those in the first class are the least harmful, but the latter cause so much harm that the community ought by some means to be able to drive them out of business."

Again he said: "The 'water cure' fakir is another quack whose titles range from 'nature cure' to 'balneotechnic.' These fakirs promise wonderful cures, but we cut short their wonderful work whenever we can. ... They are certainly criminals in every sense of the word, and while the gambler robs his victim of what he can again recover through industry and perseverance and the political mountebank may lead the people astray for awhile, the victims of medical fakirs have no chance to recover their lost health."

Very good! The last portion of the paper, as stated above, is the best. What public benefactors (?) the County Medical Societies are! But will the "honorable gentleman" explain to us why there are twenty thousand medical "quacks" at work in the city of New York? And will he also explain to us why many of them are so successful in their treatments? If he cannot, then we will endeavor to answer for him: Is it not because medicines have proven to be a failure?

When anyone becomes ill he or she usually consults a "regular" licensed physician, and after he has been experimented upon with nearly all the drugs in the Pharmacopoeia without any beneficial results he loses faith in doctors, and tries different methods of cure, as recommended by friends and acquaintances.

If physicians would not depend altogether upon drugs for curing their patients, the so-called "quack" would not exist. (Can the honorable counsel of the Medical Society contradict this statement?)

Have the members of the Society cured all the cases they have treated? How large a percentage of cures have they made? Why do two physicians of the same school contradict each other in treating the same disease? Why is it that when a sick person consults ten different physicians they will have ten different diseases and receive ten different prescriptions? Why do the best known physicians in the world prove that drugs cannot cure?

Why should protective medical laws be necessary? Of course, the honorable members of the Medical Society will say they are necessary to protect the public. But is this true? No! They have the laws passed to protect their pockets, nothing more. Medical laws would not be necessary if all physicians cured their patients.

Medicine is a false science, as proven by there being about a hundred drugs for each single ailment, and each ailment is diagnosed differently by different physicians. Why should this be so?

There are more "quacks" among the registered physicians than there are uneducated charlatans. I define a "quack" as anyone—whether a regularly educated and licensed physician or not—who takes money from another one with the promise of alleviating and curing their ailments and fails to do so. Has the Medical Society ever prosecuted a fellow member for alleged fake practice as above?

If a person has been given up as incurable by many "regular" physicians and advised to get ready to die, why should the so-called "quack," from whom the dying person derives very beneficial but unscientific (?) treatment, be branded a criminal and be prosecuted? If it is, then it is also a crime to satisfy a starving person's hunger.

The only remedy for putting the so-called medical "fakir" out of practice is for the "regular" physician to depend more upon natural remedial agents than upon drugs. He would then cure a larger percentage of cases than at present, and the public having no occasion to consult him, the "quack" would be compelled to give up housekeeping because he would have no one to cure. (*Health* magazine)

Why should protective medical laws be necessary? Of course, the honorable members of the Medical Society will say they are necessary to protect the public. But is this true? No! They have the laws passed to protect their pockets, nothing more. Medical laws would not be necessary if all physicians cured their patients.

Medicine is a false science, as proven by there being about a hundred drugs for each single ailment, and each ailment is diagnosed differently by different physicians. Why should this be so?

There are more "quacks" among the registered physicians than there are uneducated charlatans. I define a "quack" as anyone—whether a regularly educated and licensed physician or not—who takes money from another one with the promise of alleviating and curing their ailments and fails to do so. Has the Medical Society ever prosecuted a fellow member for alleged fake practice as above?

Our Medical Laws

by Benedict Lust

The Naturopath and Herald of Health, VI(6), 158-160. (1905)

In the June issue of "Health" Hugh Mann writes:
The osteopathic physicians in the State of New York are trying to have a bill passed to place the practice of osteopathy under the jurisdiction of the Board of Regents. Of course, this is being opposed by the medical societies, and during the hearing of this bill, one smart M.D., who is one of the leaders of the opposition, sprung a sensation (?) by challenging any osteopath to move one-fiftieth (1-50) of an inch the bones in a section of lamb which he exhibited.

Through this challenge the medical fraternity wanted to prove that the claims upon which osteopathy is based are false. The osteopaths by not accepting this challenge have proven themselves wise, as it is a nonsensical challenge.

The claim of the osteopaths that they can cure disease by moving the bones, and hence relieve the pressure upon nerves and ligaments, has been proven by the many remarkable and successful cures they have made. It has also been proven by the medical fraternity themselves, that in all cases of fracture of the spine the patient becomes paralyzed and when the vertebrae is replaced, thereby removing the pressure on the nerves, the patient gradually recovers. Is not this proof enough that at least some of the claims of osteopathy are correct?

If the drug doctors wish to challenge the osteopaths, or any other naturopathic physicians, why don't they do so scientifically and not theoretically? Let them choose six (6) or twelve (12) cases of three (3) or four (4) different diseases and place half of them under the care of an osteopath or other naturopath and the other half under the treatment of a representative of the M.D.'s. Let them note the results of both treatments, which should be published in one of the leading newspapers. This is the only method to prove if osteopathy or naturopathy is worthy of recognition or not. It is by their deeds we shall know them.

Before any licenses are given to the medical college graduates, they should prove that they can properly diagnose and radically cure disease. The present methods of examinations prove nothing; the graduate who has a more retentive memory will pass the examination easier than the one with a poor memory, and yet the latter may prove to be a far better physician. The theories of medical (drug) treatment are all right as far as they go, but—they do not go far enough. The public wants results and not theories.

The writer, to prove that the drugging fraternity is more in error than any branch of "Nature Cure," issues a challenge to them to answer and prove the following questions:

     I.   What is the cause of disease?

     II.   What is the cause of colds?

     III.   What is the cause of fevers?

     IV.   How is pain caused?

     V.   How do drugs cure?

     VI.   Do drugs act on living tissues, and how?

     VII.   Has medicine ever radically cured a case of epilepsy?

     VIII.   Has a case of tuberculosis of the lungs ever been cured by means of drug medication?

     IX.   Have the drug physicians ever cured a case of venereal disease, that has proven radical?

     X.   Have drugs ever cured a case of dyspepsia?

     XI.   If pneumonia, tuberculosis, smallpox, diphtheria, typhoid and scarlet fever, and other so-called infectious diseases are contagious, why do some persons become infected and others not?

The science of medicine is based on theory and not on facts. On the other hand, osteopathy, hydrotherapy, massotherapy, kinesotherapy, and other branches of naturopathy have been proven to be true therapeutic remedies by the numerous remarkable cures each single branch has accomplished.

The drug system of cure is unscientific in philosophy and practice, unreasonable in science, and contrary to the dictates of nature; it teaches a false doctrine of the action of medicines; a false doctrine of the relations of disease to the living organisms; a false doctrine of the relations of drugs to diseases; a false theory of vitality; a false theory of the remedial power of nature, and a false doctrine of "nature's law of cure."

Naturopathy is true in philosophy, harmonious with nature, and rational in practice; all of its fundamental doctrines in relation to the nature of disease, the action of remedies, the relations of diseases and remedies to each other and to the living organisms, and also in relation to vitality, the remedial power of nature, and nature's law of cure are both true and demonstrable.

All medical laws that make the drug prescribers the protectors (?) of the public, and forbid the practice of other systems of therapy, are unconstitutional and should be repealed. In place of those we should pass laws that would allow all true physicians to practice, after they had proven themselves capable of radically curing disease.

The Boards of Health should consist of three (3) practitioners of each system of therapy, and each physician who has been granted a license to practice, should be compelled to report each case he treats, and if upon a thorough investigation it is proven that a physician has neglected his proper duty, or through ignorance has failed to cure some ailment that other physicians have treated and cured, his license should be revoked. This plan would eliminate those practitioners who care more for their bank accounts, than to relive suffering, and would leave in the field the true physician who has the benefit of humanity at heart.

The drug doctor that cannot compete with the naturopath, and seeks to pass prohibitory laws, proves that he is either incompetent or lazy. If incompetent he should go into some other business, and if he is too lazy to investigate all other methods of healing, and hence be enabled to treat disease successfully, he does not deserve success, and if he starves it is his own fault.

About fifty (50) years ago Prof. R.T. Trall, M.D., in his *Water Cure Journal*, issued a challenge to the medical profession for a debate on "Nature versus Drugs." In 1901 the late Dr. August F. Reinhold also issued a challenge, that he would give $5,000 to any charitable institution, if he failed to cure any so-called incurable case that he (Dr. R.) pronounced curable. The cases to be chosen by representatives of the drug doctors. Both challenges were unheeded. If drugs cure, why don't they prove it?

Either the system of drug therapy, or naturopathy is false. That naturopathy is based on scientific and physiological facts has been proven and that the science (?) of Materia Medica is based on mere and unstable theories has also been proven; and no matter how many protective medical laws the medical societies will endeavor to pass, and how much they will oppose the recognition of naturopathy, their efforts will prove unsuccessful, because the truth can never be hidden.

> "Truth crushed to earth will rise again;
> The eternal years of 'Nature' are hers,
> But error, wounded, writhes in pain,
> And dies among his worshippers."

Since this was written the writer has received information that the osteopaths have been successful in their attempt to pass their bill. Hurrah! for truth.

Naturopathic physicians, get together.

If the drug doctors wish to challenge the osteopaths, or any other naturopathic physicians, why don't they do so scientifically and not theoretically?

All medical laws that make the drug prescribers the protectors (?) of the public, and forbid the practice of other systems of therapy, are unconstitutional and should be repealed.

1906

OPINIONS OF PHYSICIANS CONCERNING MEDICAL SCIENCE

BENEDICT LUST

———

A PLEA FOR PHYSICAL THERAPY

(*Medicine Without Medicine*)

OTTO JUETTNER, M.D., PH.D.

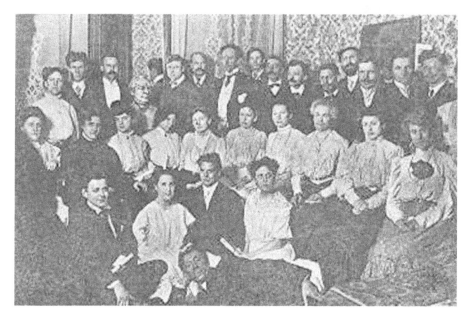

The American Naturopathic School graduating class as it appears on the cover of October, 1906, issue of *The Naturopath and Herald of Health*, Volume VII(10).

Opinions Of Physicians Concerning Medical Science

by Benedict Lust

The Naturopath and Herald of Health, VII(4), 160-161. (1906)

1. "In so-called medical science, what are accepted by authorities as indisputable facts, corroborated by proofs, are denied and refuted by other medical authorities. A kind of treatment recommended by one party as excellent is rejected by another. There are even cases where physicians will recommend processes of healing which, only a few years ago, they have condemned as detrimental to health,"—Prof. A. P. Hecker, M.D.

2. "The value of medicine is seen in the fact that in civilized countries people die more through physicians than of diseases." —Von Wedelrind, M.D.

3. "Belief in the healing power of drugs is a special product of the Middle Ages, the time of spiritual and intellectual darkness, the outcome of which was the belief in witchcraft. Luckily, the belief in witches has been overcome, but the superstition in drugs still remains. Let us try to overcome this also."—Prof. Alams, M.D.

4. "In many cases treated by physicians, chronic diseases have been subsequently brought about by the treatment of physicians." —Kieser, M.D. (System of Medicine).

5. "We have not only increased the number of diseases, but we have also made them more dangerous and more fatal." —Rusch, M.D.

6. "The idea and wish to cure patients leads medical men astray; they are like alchemists searching for the philosopher's stone." —Prof. Frerichs, M.D., Berlin.

7. "Eight-tenths of the weight of the human body consists of water, and forms the most essential part; consequently, water is the only natural drink for man. Applied externally, whether by sponge or full bath, combined with fresh air, it will prove of real blessing to the human organism."—Prof. Paesler, M.D.

8. "We must not be the least surprised at the slow success in our profession; indeed, it is only natural as long as we are not able to formulate a single sound physiological principle. I do not hesitate to state, no matter how much I wound the vanity of my colleagues, that our ignorance of the real nature of physiological disturbances of the body is so great, that it would in many cases be better not to attempt to cure at all, but to leave the case entirely to nature which, in fact, we do often enough. Even if the patient should die the sooner, we cannot state 'why' or 'wherefore' we do so, or so."—Prof. Magendie, M.D., famous French physiologist and pathologist.

9. "Our medical faculties are very narrow-minded in regard to therapeutics. They have created a dogmatism and terrorism most detrimental to the practical work of the medical profession."—Rohlfs, M.D., Goettingen,

10. "There is no science permeated with fallacies, errors, mistakes, dreams, and lies, as that of medicine."—Prof. Herm. Eberhard Richter, M.D., Dresden.

11. "Medical science with all its antiquated drugs is nothing else but a great piece of bungling."—Oesterlein, M.D.

12. "In medical science deception and illusions are far more common than in any other science, not excepting even religious superstition."—A. Foerster, M.D.

13. "Rational medical science is no longer found at our universities." —Prof. R. Virchow, M.D., Berlin.

14. "All drugs which enter the circulation of the blood, poison it in the same way as any ordinary poison which produces sickness. Drugs can never cure a disease; the latter will always be cured by nature's powers."—Prof. Smith, M.D.

15. "The inflammation of any glands may be traced to medical poison or important surgical treatment."—Prof. Gilman, M.D.

A Plea For Physical Therapy (*Medicine Without Medicine*)

by Otto Juettner, M.D., Ph.D.

The Naturopath and Herald of Health, VII(6), 225-230. (1906)

> *...and now remains*
> *That we find out the cause of this effect*
> *Or rather say, the cause of this defect,*
> *For this effect defective comes by cause.*
>
> —*Shakespeare's "Hamlet"*

It would be a most serious error to imagine that the tendency toward exactness of reasoning and toward the adoption of the so-called physiological methods of medication is a fad, like the many ephemeral notions which from time to time attracted the attention of the profession only to vanish as quickly as they have appeared. The drifting of medical thought away from the empiricism and the illusions of drug medication toward biological conceptions of disease and rational (logical, demonstrable) methods of treatment is a most characteristic sign of the times. It is but one phase in the process of evolution through which the mind of mankind has passed and is passing—not only in medicine by in all departments of human knowledge. Everywhere there is a manifest desire to inquire into the reasons of things, into the causes of the phenomena which the panorama of the living creation presents in endless number and variety. We are living in an age of inquiry. Mankind has outgrown its childhood—days when it listened in breathless suspense to fairy tales of superstition and tradition—and is loath to accept anything but what the sense reveal and the mind can see. We know that the laws of nature are necessary and eternal and that all phenomena in nature are but applications of immutable and universal principles.

The practice of medicine to-day is not what it was twenty-five years ago. The study of the natural sciences has elevated medicine to a high and dignified plane. At one time the practice of medicine was a motley mixture of notions and beliefs, almost childlike in their simplicity, and yet strangely picturesque. In medicine, and in every other branch of knowledge, things were enshrouded with that absurd mysticism that allowed no ray of light or sunshine to enter. The searcher after anatomical and physiological truth was suspected of being in truce with spirits of the regions below, and had to live in constant fear of the terrible punishment that was in store for any one who was bold enough to think. For that matter, independence of thought and action is considered a crime in some quarters even to-day. The physicians of antiquity were considered sorcerers. Their art was thought to be a sort of witchcraft, as is apparent from the word "pharmacist," which means magician. They were not really physicians in the true sense of the word. A physician, as the word indicates, is one who knows nature. They perverted nature like some people do even to-day. No wonder that Athenaeus, the historian, was rather severe in his criticism of physicians: "Exceptis medicis nil est grammaticis stultius." The curse of witchery or mysticism has clung to medicine to the present day. Human nature loves that which has an air of mystery about it. Great minds, like Boerhaave, chafed under the ballast of charlatanism that burdened the practice of medicine from the professed teachers of the healing art down to the itinerant fakir or the ignorant old woman who gathered herbs and concocted strange mixtures for the cure of every ill of the flesh.

Fingit se medicum quivis idiota profanus, Judibus, monachus, histrio, tonsor, anus.

Even at as recent a date as the fourth and fifth decades of the nineteenth century, while the seed of medical truth was being planted by great physiologists, anatomists and pathologists in Austria and Germany, there was no clinical medicine deserving of the name. The therapy taught by Schonlein, one of the most brilliant medical minds of the day, consisted in the administration of immense doses of strange and gruesome mixtures. The day of scientific medicine dawned when the master minds of the race turned to the bosom of nature as the fountainhead of all truth. The study of the natural sciences gave to mankind the elements out of which a science of medicine could be and is being constructed. It was the genius of such men as Tyndall, Darwin, Haeckl, Virchow, Helmholtz and Pettenkofer that blazed the way for truth in the interests of suffering humanity. The application of the principles gleaned from the solution of nature's mysteries has given us the system of scientific medicine, to the presentation of which, in a short and concise form, this book is devoted. The search for demonstrable truth in medicine has caused many a cherished idol of the past to tumble from its pedestal and be hopelessly shattered. If the shades of Sydenham, Hufeland and Schonlein could rise from their musty abode, they would find but a few scattered remnants of the art whose honored representatives they were in the days gone by. How true were the words of Helmholtz, spoken at a gathering in honor of that most colossal of all medical scientists of the nineteenth century, Rudolph Virchow: "Just look at Dame Medicine! You can hardly recognize the old lady since she is drinking from that fountain of youth, the natural sciences. Why, she looks so young and healthy!" What a glorious eulogy on behalf of modern clinical medicine, i. e., physiological therapeutics.

The necessary result of exact knowledge and reasoning in medicine is the dislodgement of drug-medication out of its time-honored position as the principal and essential feature of treatment. The drug idea in the treatment and cure of disease is one of those curious and unaccountable vagaries that have swayed the human mind in some manner or other from times immemorial. In the absence of knowledge, faith has ever been the anchor of hope of the human mind, even in medicine. Why the faith in the curative action of drugs taken internally should still survive among physicians is in itself a mystery as strange and singular as the lack of harmony among physicians concerning the use of drugs and the effects which are obtainable. Think of the schools, isms and pathies in medicine, of the widely divergent opinions of individual physicians concerning drugs; contemplate the drug-skepticism among doctors, which increases proportion to their experience and knowledge. There are no isms or schools in anatomy, in physiology, in physiological medication. Every physician admits without hesitation that drug-medication is uncertain and disappointing.

In spite of this it occupies the commanding therapeutic position in the colleges, in the text-books and in the sickroom. What shall the general practitioner say about drugs when men of great genius and unquestioned authority in medicine set the example of therapeutic agnosticism? Richard V. Volkmann, famed alike as a poet and a surgeon, whose splendid work in the military hospitals during the Franco-Prussian war was an inspiration to the German as well as to the French physicians who were fortunate enough to witness it, was professor at the University of Halle and second to none in point of authority. "The whole material medica," said he, in one of his lectures, "is nothing but a crude mass of empiricism. In our drug-therapy we are many times no better than the old woman and the itinerant quack—only we are 'legitimate' and they are not." Prof. Ernst Schweninger, of the University of Berlin, who was for many years the physician of Bismarck, remarked with his characteristic bluntness and candor: "One thing is certain: no really intelligent physician nowadays believes in the absurdities of drug-medication." Lauder Brunton, author of one of the best-known English books on material medica, apologizes for the lack of scientific exactness in drug-medication by referring to the latter as "an earnest and hopeful kind of empiricism." Sir Astley Cooper, the most famous English surgeon of his time, once interrupted a discussion on internal medication by saying: "No more of that! It is abominable and nauseating to think of it. The cure of disease by that sort of medication is surely a miserable make-believe." It would seem at times," opines Alonzo Clark, "that medicines have illed as many people as diseases ever did." Liebermeister, who was one of the best clinicians of his time, remarks: "How much we aim and claim to do and how very little we do accomplish!" "If all the medicines in the country were thrown in the sea," says Oliver Wendell Holmes, "it would indeed be a blessing for the people, but a trifle hard on the fishes." "Medicine," declares Rudolph Virchow, "has made rapid strides in every department except in the material medica." Scarpa and Corvisart, the physicians of the first Napoleon, admitted to the latter that "medicine is a collection of uncertain prescriptions which do more harm than good. What air, light and cleanliness cannot accomplish, no drug can do." The name of Theophrastus Paracelsus Bombastus is a synonym for quackery. At one time the bearer of the name was the most distinguished representative of the drug-therapy in Europe. History is liable to repeat itself. What appears to be a brilliant luminary to-day, may look like a dingy oil-lamp to-morrow.

The sting of hopeless skepticism has been felt by every thinking physician within his heart of hearts whenever the importance and futility of drug-treatment caused him disappointment, dissatisfaction and not infrequently humiliation. Only the young graduate who has no experience remains undaunted in his optimism. "I have ten remedies for every disease," says he, with positive assurance. After ten years of experience his optimism has given way to a sense of grim humor. "I have one remedy for ten diseases, and I am not sure of it in any of them," he is heard to remark with sorrowful emphasis. When the doctor takes sick, he is slow to take his own medicine. Individually, doctors disparage drug-treatment. Every school in medicine has its own drug-religion which is perpetuated by sectional interests and by the personal motive of the learned men who are at the head of its colleges. They all extol the exclusive virtues and truths of their own faith, while others, with equal emphasis, deride the latter and have something better of their own to offer. Forsooth, this is not an edifying spectacle for the intelligent layman to contemplate. Who is right? They cannot all be right. Perhaps they are all wrong. Even at the risk of taking that one step that is supposed to separate the sublime and the ridiculous, I cannot refrain from quoting a few humorous lines from an American medical author, who in his lighter moments wrote the following verses which convey a whole encyclopedia of therapeutic truth:

My friends, place not your faith in drugs;
They'll kill bacteria and other bugs,
If you put the medicine in their mugs,
    But this is not *de jure!*
Believe me, drugs do often lack,
But the thing that always stands to the rack

And always toes the professional crack
Is the *vis medicatrix nature!*

The HEALING POWER OF NATURE is the Alpha and Omega
of all rational therapy! To understand the motives and methods of
nature in putting this innate force to work is the beginning and the
end of medical science. To systematize our efforts in co-operating with
this universal therapeutic agent is the object of physiological therapy.
The broad basis of physiotherapy is biology, or the science which deals
with life and its manifestations. Biology is the foundation. All the natural sciences have contributed the stones out of which the stately edifice
of therapeutic truth has been constructed. Truth knows no sects. To be
a physician means to be a priest at this shrine of truth.

Has the application of abstract principles to concrete conditions established the claims of physiotherapy to clinical recognition?
We know that the ratio of recoveries from *acute diseases* is practically
the same, irrespective of drugs and schools. It seems to make no difference how much and what kind of medicine is put into a patient's
stomach, the acute disease will run its course as though nothing had
been done. Experience teaches the average physician a negative lesson. He learns what not to do. He learns the wisdom of what techni-
cally is known as the "expectant" plan of treatment. He goes through
the motions of active treatment for the benefit of the patient's relatives
and friends. The patient recovers independently of treatment; sometimes, if the doctor has not learned the negative lesson of experience,
in spite of treatment (Hughes). At times the patient does not fare quite
so well. That the chances of a patient can be lessened by meddlesome
drug-therapy, cannot be gainsaid. "One should not try to die without
medical treatment," says Moliere sarcastically. If drug-treatment were
really a necessary condition of recovery, charlatans like Dowie or the
Christian Scientists, faith-curers, etc., would have never had a hearing.
The *vis medicatrix nature* is indeed a mantle of charity that covers a
multitude of diagnostic errors and therapeutic sins. Let no one point to
the triumphs of modern medicine unless he wishes to add his testimony

to the glorious success of physiotherapeutic methods, e.g., the splendid results of hydrotherapy in typhoid fever. Even the most ardent drug dispenser will agree that the relief of a symptom now and then is all that most drugs can accomplish.

What about *chronic diseases* ? Ah, there's the rub. With a thousand or more drugs at our command, we are satisfied to give the poor sufferer a little "relief" now and then. A chronic disease is in the opinion of the great number of physicians an incurable disease. The well-informed physiotherapeutist can hold out hope long after the drug-dispenser has given up the battle. Rheumatism, neuralgia, paralysis, nervous diseases of all kinds, the thousand and one varieties of auto-intoxication, functional and reflex disorders, disease of the chest, disease of women, genitourinary and rectal disease, skin troubles, lupus, cancer, dyspepsia, constipation, in fact the whole vast army of choric diseases cannot be treated successfully without galvanism, faradism, static electricity, light frequency, X-rays, Finsen rays, Minin-rays, dry heat, vibration, massage, hydrotherapy, diet, hygienic therapy, etc.

The *utilitarian* side of the question is, last but not least, deserving of passing notice: We know that the clinical and therapeutic results in the hands of well-informed physiotherapists are necessarily better than the results of drug-treatment. The question is: Does the practice of physiological therapeutics accrue to the material, i. e., financial, benefit of the physicians who have added physiotherapy to their methods of practice? There is no class of men on earth who do as much good and receive as little in return as physicians. Of all the professions medicine is the purest and noblest, because the object of medical work is always to do good for the sake of good. Physicians are entitled to much more than they, as a class, are receiving. Philanthropic and scientific temperament does not usually go with keen commercial instincts. Hence the average physician is a poor business man. Then there is the unfair competition of the charlatan, the patent medicines, the clinics, the dispensaries, etc., etc. In addition to this it is a well-known fact that the number of physicians is increasing out all proportion to the demand. Last of all (and this is the most sententious point!), the belief in drugs is, slowly but surely, being supplanted by the belief in nature and drugless methods of medication. This and the tendency toward specialization of medical work indicate that the profession, at least as far as the general practitioner in the cities is concerned, is approaching an economic crisis, the outcome of which will be determined by the survival of the fittest. Fitness means ability to do strictly successful work.

One word more concerning the *professional* aspect of physiotherapeutic work. That the physiotherapeutist must needs be a most earnest student and a thoroughly scholarly and scientific practitioner goes without saying. This is not all that is required of him. He must be prepared to suffer from principle, to be a martyr for a good cause. He will have to face open opposition and the sling and arrows of covert adversaries. Even well-meaning friends will accuse him of ridding hobbies and of being a morbid enthusiast. His enemies in the profession will be those who are therapeutic mummies and inaccessible to new ideas of any kind. Let him find solace and inspiration in the experience of William Harvey who, almost three hundred years ago, made his immortal discovery and was rewarded by being ostracized by his colleagues, who declared that Harvey's teachings were contrary to common sense and inimical to the interests of medical practice. Then there are those who discountenance anything and everything unless it has the support of the majority of the profession. If these men could only be induced to read the history of science and particularly that of medicine, they would learn to appreciate truth for its own sake. Some of the greatest accomplishments of modern medicine can be traced to men who were not physicians at all, e. g., the ophthalmoscope, invented Helmholtz, a physicist; the principles of surgical cleanliness, first recognized by Pasteur, a chemist; the discovery of anesthetics by Morton, a dentist; the X-rays, discovered by Roentgen, a physicist; not to speak of the ignorant laymen like Brandt, Preissnitz and Schroth, who gave us the principles of gynecological massage, modern hydrotherapy and dietetics. Schiller is right when he says:

What many a wise man never sees,
Oft common sense grasps with ease.

Let the physiotherapeutist never forget that the physiological methods are the best treasures of modern medicine. Let him be a man of science in the best sense of the word. This is essential because the ubiquitous charlatan has infected the practice of modern methods with his malodorous presence. It is more especially electrotherapy and X-ray work that have suffered from the invasion of the unsavory electrical "specialist." The line of demarcation between a physician and a charlatan is that of conscience and honor. Differences of opinion concerning methods of practice or therapy do not separate those who are truly physicians. Let the legitimate practitioner rescue these glorious achievements of modern medicine out of the unclean hands of the charlatan, and thus remove the stain of quackery which physiotherapy bears in the opinion of the misinformed. Let the pioneer of the good cause push onward and upward undismayed! Let his professional work be sanctified by the knowledge that the spirit of modern medicine and the approval of the best minds in the profession are with him. Let me conclude with the epigram of Felix Niemeyer, who stated many years ago that the active principles of therapy are *Heilkraefte, nicht Heilsaefte*.

Otto Juettner
8 West Ninth St., Cincinatti, Ohio.

> *We know that the laws of nature are necessary and eternal and that all phenomena in nature are but applications of immutable and universal principles.*

1907

NEW YORK'S MEDICAL CONFRATERNITY CAUSES ARREST OF EUGENE CHRISTIAN

BENEDICT LUST

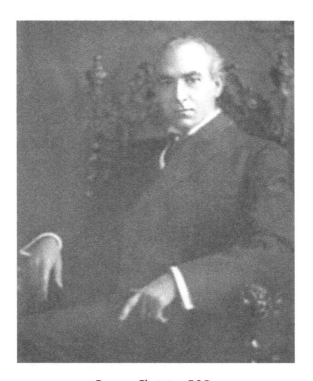

Eugene Christian, F.S.D.
Encyclopedia of Diet, Corrective Eating Society, Inc,
Vol. I, New York. (1916)

New York's Medical Confraternity Causes Arrest Of Eugene Christian

by Benedict Lust

The Naturopath and Herald of Health, VIII(5), 137-138. (1907)

Noted Dietitian Charged With Curing Human Ailments Without Drugs

The now famous case of the notorious County Medical Society of New York versus Eugene Christian, the noted food expert, has gone to the appellate division of the Supreme Court and may not be reached for several years. This case, as most readers know, is based on the charge of the drug doctors that Mr. Christian is prescribing diet for sick people without a medical license and thereby is violating the law known as the Medical Practice Act. In other words, although Mr. Christian is recognized at the present day as the greatest dietist both in this country or England, if not in the world, although he has spent years of time and study in preparation for his special work, and although he is daily curing suffering people that the drug doctors are confessedly incapable of curing, he is considered a law breaker by the medical confraternity that has brought the charge against him. Because Mr. Christian has proven the incompetency of drug doctors by accepting cases that they have pronounced "incurable" and curing them by scientific dieting, these doctors have hauled him to court as a criminal.

The charge that Mr. Christian is prescribing for the sick without a state license is merely a surface excuse for prosecuting him. There is a deeper underlying motive behind the move which was confessed to by one of the noble minded doctors who said: "The reason we are not bothering the other men in New York is because they are too small fry to bother about. We are after the big game, you know." In other words, Mr. Christian is the only man at present that the medial clique in New York fear. His position among the drugless practitioners and his phenomenal success in curing people have begun to worry the drug crowd. Moreover, as is well known, Mr. Christian is a prominent business man of New York. His close connection in this respect with the influential and well-to-do business people of the city has resulted in interesting them in his writings and in converting them away from drugs and drug doctors. Naturally, the big guns in the medical profession are alarmed. Their rich clientele is beginning to think, and confidence in drug methods is lessening appreciably. Their fees are being jeopardized. And because of these things they would like to scare Mr. Christian out of the way, but Christian don't scare a bit, and his work will go on better known than ever, besides the charge made against him is so utterly absurd that everybody laughs about it except the doctors.

Eugene Christian, through his influential social connections, is educating a class of people who, most of all, need the gospel of wholesome eating that he is preaching, but who cannot be reached by the average health reformer. Through his books on uncooked foods is due the fact that such distinguished personages as Lady Cook, Lady Dixon, Lord and Lady Beresford and others among the English nobility have become raw food enthusiasts, and the recent call to Washington, requesting him to come to the capitol to arrange an uncooked dinner for the cabinet officers and diplomatic corps, is another sign of the kind of influential people that Mr. Christian is converting to the new diet.

That Mr. Christian's growing influence is worrying the "regulars" there is not the least doubt, but when they sought to injure him by an arrest, they did not reckon with the character of the man they were attacking. In New York Eugene Christian is known as a fighter. He is a man of strong determination, and the doctors are discovering this fact now, especially in view of the fact that Mr. Christian has announced his determination to carry the case up to the highest court in the land if need be.

This stand that Mr. Christian is taking is not a personal issue affecting his business. As he said: "I can live without my professional business. In fact, my professional work is to me somewhat of a humanitarian work to which I have resolved to devote my life. But it is a vital matter of principle with me. I am fighting purely in the spirit of an American citizen, jealous of my rights, and I am going to see the ideals of American suffrage and liberty upheld."

Mr. Christian has also made it understood that his determination to take up the fight is actuated by a higher motive than regard for his own personal interests in the case. His fight will be the fight of all who are engaged in reform work. He could easily have paid the insignificant fine that might be attached to his case and gone on unmolested in his work. But that would not have helped the cause in general, and now that the doctors have begun this fight Mr. Christian proposes to end it. The issue will be decided for all time and for the benefit of all his co-workers in the cause of health reform.

The Naturopath stands in line with anybody of honest men who may set about to combat fraud in the healing arts. We say that no law can be made too stringent, no punishment too severe for that man who practices fraud in any form. But we are aware that it is not fraud that the medical societies are after. These Don Quixote efforts to protect the public are simply aimed to mislead the people. Their real purpose is to persecute those men who are rapidly supplanting them in the field of healing by using more enlightened methods of cure. All of their activity in this direction is simply a tacit acknowledgment that they cannot afford to have their antique system of drugging placed in open and fair competition with more advanced methods. They are rapidly losing public patronage and public confidence and are taking this cowardly and despicable means of stemming the tide that is turning against them. Their attempts in this direction seem to us very much like the foolish old woman of Brighton who tried to stop the rising tide with her broom.

If the dietetic treatment which Eugene Christian prescribes is not based on honest principles of cure then there is positively no occasion for the drug doctors of New York to regard him as "dangerous" to their interests. If Mr. Christian's treatment is not rational it will fail of its own account? In the final analysis of all things truth only can survive! Anything that is false, that is based on false premises, must in the end fail. This is why the drugging practice must eventually go down. We believe this to be a divine law of creation and it needs no arbitrary dictum of any set of men to say that it should be destroyed. But if his treatment is based on truth, if it is scientific, and if his methods, in fair and open competition, are able to triumph over the ideas of the old school of drug healing, then his treatment is entitled to recognition, and we assert that the men composing this political-medico clique who are trying to discredit his treatment by prosecuting him are the real criminals. They are committing a crime against God, a crime against the true progress of the healing arts, and a crime against the thousands of sick who are looking about for something other than drugs to cure them. The medical society, as it exists to-day, is organized for no higher purpose than to protect those among their crowd who are guilty of poisoning people every day in the week and they are trying to make criminals of those who are conscientiously and successfully curing patients that they are unable to cure.

Mr. Christian's fight will end with victory for him and the cause of American liberty, the same as in the Biggs case in North Carolina, and the same as in the two cases wherein the editor of this magazine was prosecuted for healing the sick without a state license. Benedict Lust was brought to trial in 1902 and also in 1904, but in both of these cases he won. Mr. Christian's fight will end just as triumphantly as those just cited. The American people are just when they stop long enough to think.

Through his books on uncooked foods is due the fact that such distinguished personages as Lady Cook, Lady Dixon, Lord and Lady Beresford and others among the English nobility have become raw food enthusiasts, and the recent call to Washington, requesting him to come to the capitol to arrange an uncooked dinner for the cabinet officers and diplomatic corps, is another sign of the kind of influential people that Mr. Christian is converting to the new diet.

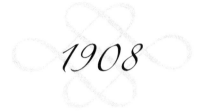

1908

Advertisement for Dr. Carl Shultz' Naturopathic establishments.

Naturopaths And Osteopaths In California

from Los Angeles Times
The Naturopath and Herald of Health, IX(1), 29-30. (1908)

For a long time a bitter fight has been waged between the Naturopaths, Osteopaths and the State Medical Board of California. While all friends of humanity and liberty hoped that Naturopathy as well as Osteopathy would be acknowledged a striking instance of the tyranny and duplicity of the political doctors has come to light. The Legislature last spring passed a new law regulating the practice of medicine in California, which law went into effect on May 1 last [1907]. This law gave the osteopaths a place on the State board, together with the allopaths, homeopaths, and eclectics. The concession was wrung from the "regulars" by the growing importance and popularity of the osteopathic schools of medicine, a school upon which the allopaths have, in the past, heaped contumely and contempt. Another school, which originated in Germany, has of late also been making great strides. The "naturopaths" include in their practice all rational methods of aiding nature to cast forth impurities from the system, such as diet, exercise, breathing, hydropathy, osteopathy, massage, electricity, etc. In this manner, remarkable cures have been effected, and it is therefore not surprising that they have brought down upon themselves the jealousy and enmity of the drug dispensers. A largely-signed petition, asking for recognition of this school, was presented to the last Legislature, and the following proposed amendment was prepared and was to be introduced by Senator McKee:

"Any person who holds a certificate from the Board of Examiners of the Naturopathic Physicians of California, elected by the Naturopathic Association of California, incorporated under the laws of this State, shall be entitled to practice Naturopathy in this State, the same as if it had been issued under this act."

On behalf of the Naturopathic Association of California the secretary, Dr. Schultz, of Los Angeles, went into communication with the State Board of Medical Examiners and also with the governor of California. For months the matter dragged along and finally the law was enacted and the Naturopaths forced out and not recognized. The last word is of course not spoken yet and as to the ultimate outcome of this controversy, there can surely be but one result. Still, as we all know, it takes time to effect reform, where we have, on the one side, "vested rights," financial interests and political influence, and, on the part of the public, ignorance and indifference.

The great importance of the subject warrants such reference. If the public fully realized the true inwardness of the medical tyranny, it would not have long to exist. It flourishes on the ignorance or the indifference of the public.

The medical trust—otherwise the American Medical Association—includes only an insignificant percentage of the practicing physicians of the United States. Yet, it has arrogated to itself the right to dictate who shall or shall not practice the healing art, in this country. It hypocritically pretends that its efforts are made for the benefit of the dear public. On the contrary, it is simply a close corporation, for the purpose of keeping out competition. If the medical trust were sincere in its declaration of interest in the welfare of the public, why has it not, long ago, started to drive out of the profession those dastardly quacks who ruin people mentally, physically and financially. These scoundrels all have diplomas, or else they could not practice.

The persecution of the medical trust is not confined to practitioners of outside schools. Worthy and able men, who have practiced their profession as M.D.'s for many years, in other States of the Union, are refused recognition in California under various specious pretexts. Some of these men, with families' dependent upon them, are today doing menial work in Southern California, because the medical trust has refused to permit them to practice their profession.

What would Americans think if it were proposed to introduce a law that only certain forms of religious worship should be permitted in this country? Yet, that is just exactly what the American Medical Association is endeavoring to do—and has, so far, to great extent been successful in accomplishing—in regard to the care of the body.

The Defense Fund

by Charles. I. White

The Naturopath and Herald of Health. IX(2), 66. (1908)

To the Drugless Healer or Physician:
I have received quite a number of letters in reply to the open letter on "The Defense Fund," published in *The Naturopath* of September last [1907].

In order that all may understand the object of "The Defense Fund" I will explain more fully. First, you all know the great medical trust, the American Medical Association, is not only doing every thing in its power to compel all sick persons to go to the M.D. and let him prescribe drugs or the knife, but it is trying in every way to drive every drugless physician out of practice, and their favorite way is to get a county attorney who will do their dirty work for them to file a complaint against the drugless doctor in the county court. The M.D. will furnish a witness, or several of them, who will swear to such things as they are told to say, and you are bound over. Right here comes the great point: Not one drugless doctor in a hundred has funds enough to defend himself and take his case to the State Supreme Court if he is beaten in the district or county court. If it was known that the defendant had funds to take his case up and stay with it, the county attorney would think at least twice before he filed the complaint, as the county might lose the case. There is not one case in a hundred that will come down from the Supreme Court as it went to it, but will come back as the Dr. Biggs case of North Carolina, in favor of drugless healing.

Now in regard to "The Defense Fund," Benedict Lust, N.D., president of the Naturopathic Society of America, and publisher of *The Naturopath*, Magazine, will receive and receipt for money sent him to apply to the Defense Fund. The amount subscribed to the Defense Fund, along with the names of each subscriber, will be published in *The Naturopath* each month. I believe the Naturopathic Society of America to be the banner under which we drugless physicians can and will become free from the prosecutions of the political M.D.

We never know just when we will be "next" to be arrested and put to a great expense and trouble as things are to-day.

During sixteen years of drugless healing I have been arrested nine times and put under bonds, but I can truthfully say that there never has been any complaint filed by a patient, but in each case the arrest was caused and brought about by an M.D. The last case in which I was convicted in the district court at Grand Island, Neb., was a big farce. I was convicted on the evidence of one man, and that man swore to a lie. If this case had been taken through the State Supreme Court the result would have been a victory for the drugless dealer, but the case had cost me over $200 and I did not have the funds to take it through the Supreme Court. A Defense Fund would have changed things in the State of Nebraska. As it is, every drugless doctor or healer runs a chance of being arrested just as soon as he becomes a little successful. It is the same old story and you all know it.

Now why not get free? We can do so. Once it becomes known that we have ample funds to defend our rights we will be let alone. Think hard, but think quick, and then act promptly as you think best, not only for your own good, but for the good of all. Write Benedict Lust, N.D., 124 E. 59th St., New York City, send him $5 to apply to the Defense Fund account, and request him to explain the workings of the proposition, etc., and DO IT NOW.

I would be glad to receive letters on this subject from all who care to write me. My only interest in the Defense Fund is to push it along, as I believe it to be a good thing.

Yours for the Defense Fund,

Dr. Chas. I. White
865 10th St., Riverside, Cal.

BERNARR MACFADDEN

by Benedict Lust

The Naturopath and Herald of Health. IX(3), 98. (1908)

Last November Bernarr Macfadden, well known editor of the *Physical Culture Magazine* and the champion of the physical movement in this country, was convicted for publishing articles and stories in his magazine which were intended for a better education and enlightenment, showing also the demoralization of our people at large. Instead of finding encouragement and endorsement for warning the public from such dangers he was persecuted by the National Purity Association through its representative, Anthony Comstock, and was convicted. The judgment was a fine of $2,000 and two years in the penitentiary at hard labor. This whole persecution of Macfadden finds its source in the medical trust which tries to undermine and weed out every movement which stands for enlightenment along the physiological methods. The doctors, especially those who belong to the medical association, are determined to keep the public in the dark and to suppress all literature which would educate the people of the dangers of medical treatment, vaccination and other superstitions along these lines. Undoubtedly Macfadden has become the victim of these forces who worked in the dark. We sympathize with him. Macfadden has exposed degeneracy as it exists in all its manifold ways in American life. He is a road breaker and deserves gratitude, co-operation and good will of every practicing naturopath, of the nature cure societies, and every man and woman who believes and stands for truth, regeneration and natural ways of living and healing. Macfadden had not given up yet and has appealed to Washington for another trial. At the same time lists are circulating to get signatures and to submit a petition of at least one million subscribers for a pardon of B. Macfadden. I am sure if this matter is fully submitted to Theodore Roosevelt that he will reverse the judgment. We are requesting all our readers to sign these petitions and write to Mr. Macfadden, Flatiron Building, New York, for petition blanks and for literature on this case. Blank forms can also be had from our office, and friends of B. Macfadden who come in here can also sign such petitions here which will be forwarded to the proper place.

It is a pity that in this advanced age of enlightenment people can be found who will stand up against a man like Macfadden. The jury instead of reading the whole story only convicted him for one sentence. The connection with it was not read and studied. The judge told the jury he would like to see Macfadden convicted and so they convicted him. But we know Macfadden too well, and he will not give up. I am sure he will come out triumphantly, and that will be of benefit to the whole movement of natural healing and living. Brother Macfadden deserves the sympathy and co-operation of every reader of this magazine.

> *The judgment was a fine of $2,000 and two years in the penitentiary at hard labor. This whole persecution of Macfadden finds its source in the medical trust which tries to undermine and weed out every movement which stands for enlightenment along the physiological methods. The doctors, especially those who belong to the medical association, are determined to keep the public in the dark and to suppress all literature which would educate the people of the dangers of medical treatment, vaccination and other superstitions along these lines.*

Another Medical Persecution

by Benedict Lust

The Naturopath and Herald of Health. IX(6), 190-191. (1908)

The latest move of the medical trust in Los Angeles has been to cause the arrest of Dr. Carl Shultz of South Hope Street on a charge of practicing medicine without a license.

For a number of years Dr. Schultz has conducted a modest nature cure sanatorium in this city, aided by his wife, who is also experienced in treating human ills. He gives no drugs, using only natural methods, such as mav[sic] aid nature to cast forth impurities—methods that are employed in leading nature-cure establishments in the United States and Europe, such, for instance, as massage, osteopathy, hydropathy and diet, the latter being strictly vegetarian. His place is clean and home-like. Dr. Shultz is a hard worker and thoroughly conscientious, who takes far more than a financial interest in his allotted task of aiding sick people to get well, and keep well. Such an occupation is an exhausting one. Your conscientious osteopath, or naturopath, has a far different job from the allopath, who merely taps on your chest, and writes out a prescription. It is hard work, mentally and physically, and is made more so by the fact that people rarely resort to the natural method of cure, which involves self-denial, until they have exhausted every other medical device, and have been given up as hopeless by the "regulars".

The specific charge upon which Dr. Schultz was arrested is that he cared at his establishment for a man and wife who under his treatment recovered their health, although they had been considered hopeless cases. They were poor people, and had no money to pay for the treatment, in consequence of which Dr. Shultz accepted a note for half the regular charge, or about enough to pay for modest board and lodging. The real cause for his arrest is the fact that, first, he has been doing people good physically, and this interferes with the business of the profession, and secondly, that he has incurred the enmity of one of the members of the State board by exposing, some months ago, in the columns of this department, the duplicity of that member, when the medical bill was before the last Legislature.

Dr. Schultz has diplomas from two osteopathic colleges, outside of California. The local osteopaths will, however, not permit him to graduate here, for the reason that he uses other methods besides osteopathy, and is therefore not ethical. This shows that some of the osteopaths are becoming as narrow in their views as the "regulars."

The old saying, "whom the gods wish to destroy they first make mad," may appropriately be quoted here. One would suppose that the medical trust would "lay low," for a time, after the snub it got from the Supreme Court of New York for causing the arrest of Eugene Christian because he had been guilty of the heinous crime of teaching people to eat raw food. Meantime, as we have frequently pointed out, while they are persecuting and prosecuting honest men, they fail absolutely to take any step whatever against the scores of scoundrel quacks who prostitute their profession, and ruin people, physically and financially. Why is this? Simply because these fellows all have an M.D. diploma hanging in their offices. Therefore, they are immune. Surely, a medical diploma, like charity, covers a multitude of sins.

The medical inquisitors claim that they are unable to reach these medical fakers, because they have diplomas, and are thus protected by the law. If so, it is sufficient to say that the law is a miserable farce. But it is not so. At least, it is not so in New York State, where the County Medical Society recently issued a pamphlet showing a long list of quacks that had been convicted in the Court of Special Sessions of the first division of New York, including "specialists for men," abortionists, fake magnetic curers, and others. Yet, this same society caused, through detectives, the arrest of a worthy man, Eugene Christian, because he instructed people in regard to diet. Thus, they showed plainly that these medical laws are not, as they claim, for the protection of the people, but for the perpetuation of the medical trust, which is as proscriptive, tyrannical and unreasonable as the San Francisco plumbers' union.

How long this un-American condition of affairs shall be allowed to prevail rests upon the American people. They are beginning to realize the fact that it is as unreasonable and unjust to force a man to accept any one particular kind of medical treatment as it would be to force him to worship in the church of one particular sect. Especially is this true in view of the fact of the dismal failure of medical "science," so-called, to succeed in restoring the sick to health.

Dr. Schultz will fight the case, and, if necessary, carry it to the Supreme Court.

—Los Angeles Times.

The specific charge upon which Dr. Schultz was arrested is that he cared at his establishment for a man and wife who under his treatment recovered their health, although they had been considered hopeless cases.

REMOVAL NOTICE

by Benedict Lust

The Naturopath and Herald of Health, IX(12), 367. (1908)

It gives me great pleasure to announce that we have succeeded in finding better and larger quarters for our Naturopathic Sanitarium in New York as well as for our Publishing Department. On or about December 15th, we will move anything and everything, the store included, to the building at No. 465 Lexington Avenue, between Forty-fifth and Forty-sixth Streets, where everything in the future will be transacted. The basement will be fitted up for the store and for the publishing office and on the first floor will be the parlor, lecture hall, dining room, treatment rooms for the outside patients, and a general office. The three other floors will be used for patients who stay in the house. The top floor is arranged for the American School of Naturopathy. Fine class rooms, gymnasium, all appliances for the practical demonstration of Naturopathy and a number of rooms to be rented out with or without board, to the students.

At this building are facilities for 100 guests. We will also receive boarders and transient guests. The table will be strictly naturopathic-vegetarian, and transients can have rooms and board by the day or week and also single meals at a reasonable price. This house will answer the purpose in every respect. The location is most excellent, right near the Grand Central Depot, only three blocks from the elevated railroad, subway and Forty-second Street. The house is open on three sides, facing a beautiful private park, and every room has sunshine and plenty of light. The house has all modern improvements, steam heating, electric light, elevator service, porch, etc. We invite all our old and new friends to call and inspect the new headquarters.

1909

The Naturopathic Society of America [N. S. A.] had regular informative meetings for its members.

A Family Chat Concerning Our Growth

by Benedict Lust

The Naturopath and Herald of Health, XIV(1), 1-2. (1909)

I don't believe much in looking backward—the people who do it have finished their work. Our work is just begun, although we've been at it fourteen years with every year more strenuous than the one before. But the mother of a family can't help noticing how finely her children are growing; and this Parent Institution of Naturopathy is delighted with the progress of her offspring throughout America.

Not so long ago, I remember how the **orthodox** heretics in the Healing Brotherhood—there are many such—objected to the name, misunderstood the purpose, and doubted the ultimate success of Naturopathy. They said we were bound to fail unless we adopted a fad of some kind, sold a high-priced remedy or machine, followed the patent medicine style of advertising, catered to fanatics, or otherwise fooled the people and betrayed our own ideals.

Today, many of our early critics have themselves gone to the wall, a few are struggling to exist on a half-charity basis, and the **successful ones have either patterned their methods after ours or acknowledge the supremacy of our ideas by taking them bodily.** The word "Naturopathy" is familiar to health-seekers from the Atlantic to the Pacific, from the Gulf of Mexico to the Alaskan boundaries, on the Eastern Hemisphere and even in the Islands of the sea. Practitioners we never heard of are signing "N.D." to their names---and there's no better proof of success than to be widely imitated. Articles, editorials and opinions from this magazine we find reprinted in many of the high-class publications. Our graduates have established themselves all over this country—some of them have already won a national reputation.

You can afford to be proud, sister and brother readers, of your connection with the greatest Health movement in the world's whole experience. They're all coming—the "specialists" who imagined they had possession of Truth when they only observed one side of Truth from a distance. New Thought magazines run departments of Diet, Exercise, Breathing and Baths, wide-awake churches conduct regular clinics in the gospel of Health. Osteopaths and Physical Culturists include mental attitude as a necessary factor, and **everybody who grows must grow Naturopathic.**

The American School of Naturopathy has approximately 500 graduates to its credit since 1901, the year of its founding. The second institution, that maintained in Los Angeles, under the wise and skillful direction of Dr. Carl Schultz, numbers about 200 graduates in four years of service. The third great school, established more recently by Dr. Lindlahr in Chicago, has been phenomenally successful; I don't know just how many students it has qualified, but I do know how good. Dr. Lindlahr's hold on people of wealth and refinement is very exceptional in the ranks of Natural Healing.

There are upwards of 2,000 practicing Naturopaths in America today. Ten years ago there were less than a hundred. When you consider that each of these Naturists is a teacher no less than a healer, a radiating centre[sic] of influence through the community, you get some idea of how fast we're growing.

The fourth Naturopathic college will probably arise in Texas. Negotiations are under way at the present time. Texas is miraculously populated with **doctors who think.** Result: the old school and the new school play in each other's yard when their patients aren't looking, thus picking up and taking home many a stray bit of useful information.

Two publications were born in 1908, and right heartily we welcome them to our family. Dr. Lindlahr's *Nature Cure Magazine* and Rev. Johannes *Glaesser's Deutch-Amerikanisher Natur-Artz* belong on your study-table alongside *The Naturopath.* One of the greatest helps to the individual lies in comparing the different interpretations of Naturism. Your instinct may tell you to do the exact opposite of what my instinct tells me. And if you study the various conclusions of those who follow **their** instinct, you'll be able to discover which way **yours** leads—and you'll do it a lot quicker.

A recent example of **European science** combined with **American**

push is the splendid work of Dr. MacGregor Reid, No. 57 Fleet Street, London. His Nature Cure Magazine has taken first place among its older brethren in a wonderfully short time. And the chain of societies he has formed extending all over Great Britain has a parallel nowhere but in the life of Father Kneipp, whose mission to Germany antedated that of Dr. Reid to England.

In line with the Naturopathic policy of enlargement, we are making an important change for the New Year. After January 1st you will find us on Lexington Avenue. Please jot it down for reference. This house is just the one we've been looking for. Situated on a quiet street, with sunlight flooding three sides, and overlooking a beautiful garden, the residence was formerly used as a Health Home and therefore suits our purpose admirably. We'll tell you more about it later. Meanwhile the latch-string is always out, and we shall be glad to see you as a visitor, patient, student, friend, or inquirer.

Practitioners we never heard of are signing "N.D." to their names—and there's no better proof of success than to be widely imitated. Articles, editorials and opinions from this magazine we find reprinted in many of the high-class publications. Our graduates have established themselves all over this country—some of them have already won a national reputation.

The American School of Naturopathy has approximately 500 graduates to its credit since 1901, the year of its founding.

OUR NEW NATUROPATHIC HOSPITAL

by Benedict Lust
The Naturopath and Herald of Health, XIV(2), 87-89. (1909)

This is an open Letter to our Readers, a heart-to-heart unfolding of a long cherished plan to make Naturopathy the standard system of Healing and Living in the great centres of population. I do not think any matter of so great importance has ever been brought to your attention, and I am sure you will wish, as loyal Naturopaths, to give it your special consideration.

During the past thirteen years of practical work in drugless therapeutics, the editor of this magazine has had thousands of requests from people all over the world who believed in our methods yet could not afford the time or money for personal treatment.

Literally, hundreds of deserving cases have been turned away from our Health Home, simply because we lacked facilities to do this work on a large scale and a purely philanthropic basis. In spite of great financial burdens and difficulties, we have done all we could to relieve suffering without pay—many a touching letter of gratitude comes to this office and is at once destroyed. Until you have been in such a position as ours you can have no idea how pitiful it is to realize the number of human wrecks that the druggist, the doctor, and the surgeon have made—and left to die.

One of the awful injustices of America, so-called free, is that **the poor are absolutely at the mercy of the doctors.** Hospitals are favored by municipalities because giving to frivolous medical students and bungling interns a chance to witness the latest experiment in scientific carving. The **feelings of the patient** are never considered—unless to be recorded as unique psychological data. "Lie down and die, that we may observe the process," this is the highly civilized thought uppermost in that vacancy called a mind, owned by the average hospital attendant. A century from now, the "regular" therapeutic methods of today will seem as barbarous as blood-letting and Voodoo-craft appear to us.

All modern thinkers are aware of the superstition, criminal guess-work and utter lack of reason in the usual hospital procedure. More often than the outside world imagines, the operator deliberately cuts a patient open to find out what ails the man—we have known many such cases. Intentional cruelty is practiced where least suspected; a number of exposures in the newspapers of this city have revealed a hideous condition throughout certain prominent hospitals and asylums; guarded by the secrecy of medical practice, half-grown employees are allowed to maltreat the aged and infirm with a degree of brutality too heart-breaking for a description. In even the best hospitals the usual atrocities practiced on women and girls are enough to make a fiend blush with shame, that creatures in the form of men should be so lacking in manliness. How can the body be reverenced as the temple of the spirit by those whose one aim is to mutilate the body?

The anxiety cause by ignorant diagnosis; the misery of needless operations; the risk of life and happiness at the hands of a clumsy tinker endeavoring to improve on Nature; the embarrassment of hasty exposure and rough examinations; the loss of time and waste of money while recovering from the surgeon's mistake; the atmosphere of poisons and phantoms of death that commonly fill a sick-room known as a public ward; the total indifference to human life and irresponsibility in handling it; these are a few of the wretched marks of a hospital that make the average person prefer to run the risk of an easier death at home. This is a sad condition of affairs, that the one place on earth which is meant to soothe, cheer, and comfort should only add to the burden of physical suffering a heavier one of mental anguish.

A rich and prominent man of Brooklyn was recently bitten by a pet dog. Expensive doctors prophesied hydrophobia, and hurried the unfortunate to a sterilizing institution lauded by medical science. Shortly the man died in convulsions, whether from the fear **created by the doctors,** or from the treatment administered by them, none can say. Many of the world's most useful citizens, from President McKinley down, have been literally slain by those employed to heal them. Isn't it time for a Hospital founded on common-sense?

What this country needs most is a **practical** demonstration of Naturopathy on a large scale—an institution corresponding to that of Bilz, Kneipp, or Lahmann or Just, where the great masses of the people may come and be healed, then go forth and tell their friends. Every large city could easily support a wisely directed Home of Natural Healing. New York, for example, has a number of charity concerns so richly endowed that their management is at a loss how to spend the money. Yet one Naturopathic Hospital would be more valuable to the community than a score of the old-fashioned kind.

Ever since the founding of the Naturopathic Institute we have had in mind the opening of a **Hospital which must also be the School of Natural Living.** The demand for this has grown so tremendously of late that we are impelled to act at once. Hence this letter to you, who are interested the same as ourselves. The Hospital idea we have submitted to more than 500 friends of the cause. They are all enthusiastic. They are not rich people—except in friendliness, sympathy, and good-will. Most of them are plain German or German-American citizens of only moderate means, but **willing to do what they can.** And if all our readers have that spirit, this Hospital will be going in a very short while.

An association has been organized for establishing and maintaining Naturopathic Hospitals and Schools. A governing Board of Ten is composed of well-known business and professional men, who will administer affairs in a manner wholly unprejudiced and far-seeing. The Hospital Association will never be connected with any private enterprise. The Hospital Fund will be so invested that not a penny can be used for any other purpose than the one specified. Subscriptions and donations will be recorded month by month in THE NATUROPATH; also as personal receipt will be mailed as a legal guarantee.

Every charitable institution should become self-supporting. This will, in the course of time. But for the start, the movement depends entirely on the voluntary subscriptions of those who believe in the work. The list of pledges begins thus:

Benedict Lust, N. D., 465 Lexington Av., N. Y...........$1,000
Theobald Schaibly, 343 Broadway, Brooklyn, N. Y......... 100
Jakob Reidmüller, N. D., 117 E. 86th St., N. Y...............100

Louis Lust, 100 E. 105th St., N. Y............................ 100
The Naturopathic Society of America, Section N. Y...... 100
Naturheilverein "Kneipp," N. Y. City....................... 100

Together to Feb. 1st, 1909................................ $1,500

If there ever was a noble charity, or ever will be, could any compare with this? It is to be the first great institution in American where the common people may not only be healed of their afflictions, but will also be taught how never to be sick again. They need not even stop work; in most cases one daily treatment, with full instructions as to diet, baths, exercise, et cetera, will ensure complete recovery and a new-found happiness.

This is to be a cheerful place, where **Life** is always in the mind, heart and body—instead of things dead and dying. The spirit will be uplifting, the labor performed in love and sympathy, the feeling of human brotherhood made to supplant all theories about disease. We believe with Kuhne that "Only cleanliness heals." So our Hospital won't contain ill-smelling bottles intended to drown something worse— it will show clean everywhere, clean physically, mentally and morally. Neither shall we tolerate graft in the management—we shall keep the books open for any one's inspection, and thank you for your interest.

All natural practitioners know how quickly most ailments are relieved by the simple use of air-baths, hot or cold water treatments, massage, regulation of diet, scientific deep breathing, and confident statements of perfect health. The Naturopathic Hospital will first show people how this is done—then instruct them how to do it for themselves until such time as disease will be routed from their lives. Plenty of buildings are to be had which a very little re-modeling would make finely suitable; and where educational classes may be conducted apart from the healing rooms. One such house we have particularly in view, to be secured the moment that the funds warrant us in going ahead.

We need not assure you that drugs will be absent, and operations limited to accidental or last-resort cases. You know what a model institution such as we are planning will have to be—and it will be that as soon as you help us get it started. Once **we prove what Naturopathy has done** for the sick and miserable of the world, plenty of rich folks will come with regular donations. But every dollar given to-day will be **a stone in the foundation**—the dollars that are offered to-morrow may buy only pictures for the walls.

We have hundreds of letters on file from students and patients who wished to express their gratitude in some tangible way. This is the way. And now is the time—a very little co-operation from every single reader **at the beginning** will prove more valuable than million-dollar gifts can do ten years from now.

Ask for more particulars; write us or come in and talk things over. Make suggestions, offer criticisms, do anything to let us know you are interested and want to help.

Here is a vital point. If you cannot afford to send cash at once, then just sign your pledge for the amount and mail that for deposit. We will notify you when the money will be actually needed. Cash is better, since it draws interest. But **response** of any kind is good, and your promise is enough.

Another thing. Don't hesitate because your gift looks small. If you are modest about it, we won't publish your name in the Monthly Bulletin. But we would rather have a hundred $1.00 subscriptions than a single $1,000 offer; because the moral support and mental encouragement of a hundred individuals will advance the work more than anybody's lump of gold possibly could. Checks should be written payable to **The Naturopath, Account Hospital Fund,** 465 Lexington Av., N. Y. City.

Naturopathy Legalized In California

by Benedict Lust
The Naturopath and Herald of Health, XIV(3), 183-185. (1909)

D r. Carl Schultz, of Los Angeles, who recently returned from Sacramento, brought the important information that the bill licensing naturopathy had passed both houses of the Legislature. The Governor has since signed the bill. Dr. Schultz and his good wife have worked indefatigably for years for such a measure as this. California is now in line with Germany, where the "nature cure" has held a high position for more than half a century, where the "nature cure" has held a high position for more than half a century.

The bill referred to is "Committee Substitute for Senate Bill No. 26." It was introduced by the Committee on Public Health and Quarantine, on February 24. It is entitled: "An Act to Amend Section Sixteen of an Act Entitled 'An Act for the Regulation of Practice of Medicine and Surgery, Osteopathy, and Other Systems or Modes of Treating the Sick or Afflicted in the State of California, and for the Appointment of a Board of Medical Examiners in the Matter of Said Regulation.' (Approved March 14, 1907.)"

Following is a copy of the bill:

"Section I. Section 16 of an act entitled 'An act for the regulation of the practice of medicine and surgery, osteopathy, and other systems or modes of treating the sick or afflicted, in the State of California, and for the appointment of a board of medical examiners in the matter of said regulation,' approved March 14, 1907, is amended to read as follows:

"Section 16. Any person who holds a certificate from the Board of Medical Examiners created by 'An act for the regulation of the practice of medicines and surgery in the State of California, and for the appointment of a board of medical examiners in the matter of such regulation,' which took effect August the first, 1901, or from one of the boards of examiners heretofore existing, under the provisions of 'An act to regulate the practice of medicine in the State of California,' approved April

3, 1876, or an act supplemental and amendatory to said act, which became a law April 1, 1878, shall be entitled to practice medicine and surgery in this State, the same as if it had been issued under this act; any person who holds a certificate from the Board of Osteopathic Examiners of the State of California, under the provisions of 'An act to regulate the practice of osteopathy in the State of California, and to provide for a State Board of Osteopathic Examiners, and to license osteopaths to practice in this State, and to punish persons violating the provisions of this act,' which became law under constitutional provisions, without the Governor's approval, March 9, 1901, shall be entitled to practice osteopathy in this State, the same as if it had been issued under this act. Any person who holds an unrevoked certificate issued by the board of examiners of the Association of Naturopaths of California, incorporated under the laws of the State of California, August 8, 1904, and who shall be practicing naturopathy prior to the passage of this act, shall be entitled to practice naturopathy in this State, the same as if it had been issued under this act. The Board of Medical Examiners shall endorse said certificate at their first meeting after this act becomes a law, or at any subsequent meeting after this act becomes a law, or at any subsequent meeting of the board, but not later than six months after the passage of this act, by signature of its president and secretary and affixing its official seal. Provided, however, that the holder of such certificate has signed his or her name on the back of said certificate and president and secretary of the Association of Naturopaths of California, have certified over their respective signatures that the holder of said certificate is the rightful owner of same. But all certificates herein mentioned may be revoked for any unprofessional conduct, in the same manner and upon the same grounds as if they had been issued under this act.

"Sec. 2. This act shall take effect and be in force from and after its passage."

—*Los Angeles Times.*

Naturopaths In Oregon

by P. T. Ball

The Naturopath and Herald of Health, XIV(4), 190. (1909)

We received the following communication on March 12th from Dr. Phillip T. Ball, 616 Rothschild Bldg., Portland, Ore.:

Our association is on a sound footing now, and we have defeated the obnoxious law that the medical doctors tried to get through the Legislature, which was intended to put everybody out of business but themselves in the business of healing the sick. We are trying to get a law passed making the Naturopaths legal practitioners. As it is, we have got a clause tacked onto the law that the Osteopaths got through exempting us and the Chiropractors from the provisions of their bill. We have paid all our expenses of sending a deputation to Salem to see the senators and explain the result of the law like the medical doctors wished to get through, and we have incorporated under the State laws, and our officers are as follows:

President, Dr. W. E. Mallory.
First Vice President, Dr. I. H. Howard.
Second Vice President, Dr. J.N. Dunn.
Treasurer, Dr. A. Bertschinger.
Secretary, Dr. Phillip T. Ball.

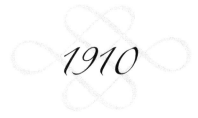

1910

The Anti-Vaccine Crusade

Henry Lindlahr, M.D.

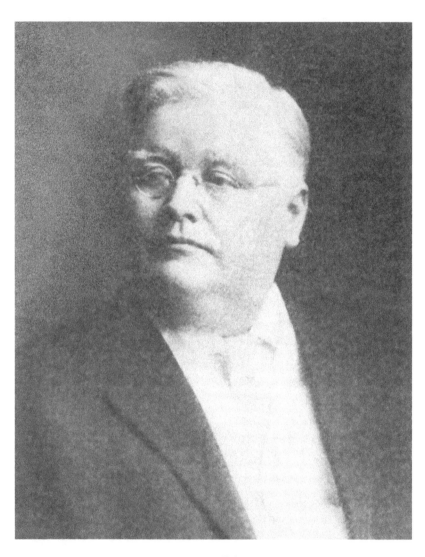

Dr. Henry Lindlahr, M.D.

THE ANTI-VACCINE CRUSADE

by Henry Lindlahr, M.D.

The Naturopath and Herald of Health, XV(3), 129-132. (1910)

"To vaccinate or not to vaccinate," that is the question of the day in Chicago.

In order to solve this much discussed problem intelligently and rationally it becomes necessary to understand the true nature of acute and chronic diseases.

Modern "regular" medical science is built on the germ theory of disease. The microscope discloses to the astonished eye of science the wonders of the world of micro-organisms. Many forms of disease are found to be accompanied by the production of certain kinds of germs, bacteria, and parasites.

In malarial diseases we find in the blood in great numbers of the **plasmodium malariae**; in cholera, the cholera bacillus; in consumption, the tubercle bacillus, etc., and forthwith scientists argue that these germs are the true causes of disease. As a natural corollary to this assumption they further conclude that in order to cure the disease they must kill the germs.

From these premises have evolved our modern theory and practice of medicine and surgery, culminating in the lymph, serum, vaccine, and antitoxin therapy.

Kill the bug and cure the disease, that sounds possible—but is it true?

Only a few years ago the world was all aglow with excitement over Dr. Koch's wonderful discovery, and he was heralded as one of the great figures of humanity. He claimed that the tubercle bacillus was the cause of consumption, and that his tuberculin, a decoction of tubercle bacilli, was certain death to the bacilli and a sure cure for consumption. The German Parliament, in the first excitement over the wonderful discovery, presented to him in the name of the nation a vote of thanks, and the sum of 100,000 marks.

From all parts of the world consumptives and those who were in dread of becoming such came to try the new treatment. But, alas, to-day tuberculin is almost forgotten. Only here and there a lone fakir poses as the original Dr. Koch from Berlin, and sells to poor deluded sufferers the wonderful tuberculin as a sure cure for consumption, and in Berlin people show you "Koch's graveyard," where lie buried thousands of victims of tuberculin.

Like the tuberculin and like many another **ignis fatuus** of medical science, every other form of lymph, serum, vaccine, and antitoxin will also in time sink into merited oblivion. Health can never be created by putting viral poisons into the human body.

Naturopathy holds that germs, bacteria and parasites are products of disease rather than its cause. The sugar solution may create yeast germs, but yeast germs cannot create a sugar solution. Disease matter in the body, as we shall see, corresponds to the sugar in a fermenting fluid.

Which is the more probable, that foul air, filth, and dirt create fungi and vermin in a house, or that the fungi and vermin create the foul air, dirt, and filth? Is it not evident that medical science has put the cart before the horse?

What would the learned professor of bacteriology say if some day he found his trusted Bridget going through the house with a carbolic acid sprinkler trying to extirpate dirt and microbes, instead of using a goodly supply of soap, water, fresh air and sunlight?

Cleanliness inside and out, in the body, the home, the street and the alley, is the only rational preventative and cure of infectious, bacterial and parasitic diseases.

Naturopathy claims that germs of themselves alone cannot create disease—if they could, humanity would soon be extinct. Disease germs are present everywhere, on the food we eat, and the water we drink, and air and dust we breathe, and on the money we handle. Can you imagine anything fouler and more thoroughly saturated with disease germs and bacteria than our beloved money? Has it not been passed through thousands of dirty pockets and diseased hands? But that does not deter the most delicate lady and the most rabid bacteria crank from fondling it—but—"be sure and boil the water." To be consistent why not disinfect our greenbacks?

Why not wear filter before nose and mouth when shopping downtown among holiday crowds? Oh, Sancta Simplicitas, just think of it— we cannot spend fifteen minutes in such a surging, perspiring mass of humanity without inhaling in the foul air and dust every disease germ in existence; why then do not all the people lay down and die? Because it takes something more in the system than microbes to create disease, namely, lowered vitality and morbid matter; in other words—the disease predisposition. These factors given, the conditions are ripe for the development of germ diseases.

Just as yeast grows in a sugar solution only, so grow and multiply disease germs in disease matter only. Yeast germs will not grow and multiply in clear water because they find no nourishment, nor will disease germs grow and multiply in pure blood and normal tissues in a body possessed of good vitality. They find nothing to subsist upon. The vigorous, vibratory activity of a healthy organism repels and eliminates the invaders without much trouble. These dreaded and maligned little invaders are not nearly so black as painted by medical science; indeed, under certain circumstances, they become our best friends.

They are, in most instances, nothing more or less to nature's scavengers, and to destroy them would be about as sensible as to kill the "white angels" of our street cleaning brigades, who in the performance of their duty are compelled to stir up the dust and dirt.

Fevers and inflammations in the human organisms are closely related to the process of fermentation. Every housewife is familiar with the phenomenon of fermentation. When yeast is added to the saccharine solution, grape juice for instance, a great activity ensues, bubbles arise, the fluid is agitated in violent commotion, the temperature increases, scum forms on the surface, and the sediment at the bottom. If this activity is allowed to continue unhindered, yeast germs, while digesting it, split up the grape sugar into alcohol and carbonic acid. When all the sugar has been thus removed and transformed, the resultant is a fluid of crystalline clearness which we call wine.

The process of fermentation, however, can be arrested at any time by the addition of salicylic acid, formaldehyde, or any other powerful antiseptic. But what happens? If the fermentation is thus suddenly arrested the resulting fluid contains a mass of unfermented sugar, dead yeast germs, and poisonous antiseptics. It has become a nasty, torpid mass, repulsive to sight, smell and taste. In this we have a perfect simile of the **modus operandi** of acute and chronic diseases and their treatment.

When disease germs find in the human body the necessary conditions for growth and propagation—namely, lowered vitality, and their own congenial morbid soil—they multiply very rapidly and develop all the symptoms of that particular germ disease. Similar to the phenomenon of fermentation we observe accelerated circulation, rapid pulse, increased temperature, congestion, and quickened elimination in the form of mucus, pus, perspiration, and other morbid discharges.

The greatly increased vital activity in the system indicates simply that nature, by means of germs, parasites, and fever heat is endeavoring to stir up, consume, and eliminate from the system waste and morbid matter.

If these processes of elimination are allowed to run their course in a natural manner, and when purification and elimination are fully completed, the acute symptoms will subside of their own accord, and after such a "natural cure" the patient is actually rejuvenated, and says that he feels like a "new man."

As in the case of alcoholic fermentation it is an easy matter to arrest by antiseptics, antipyretics, and germicides the process of fever and inflammation, but what is the result? Nature is thwarted in her attempt to burn up and eliminate the waste and morbid matter from the system. Drug poisons are added to disease poisons and as a result nature's acute healing and cleansing efforts are turned into latent chronic diseases.

To quote from our *NATUROPATH* Series: "When unnatural habits of life, before alluded to, have lowered the vitality and favored the accumulation of waste matter and poisons to such an extent that the sluggish bowels, kidneys, skin and other organs of elimination are unable to keep a clean house, nature has to resort to other more radical means of purification or **we would choke in our own impurities.** These forcible house cleanings of nature are fevers, catarrh, skin eruptions, diarrheas, boils, abnormal perspirations, and many other so-called 'acute diseases.' Sulphur and mercury may drive back the skin eruptions; antipyretics and antiseptics may suppress fever and catarrh. The patient and the doctor may congratulate themselves on the speedy cure, but what is the true state of affairs? Nature has been thwarted in her work of healing and cleansing. She had to give up the fight against disease matter in order to combat the more potent poisons of mercury, quinine, iodine, strychnine, or whatever they may be termed.

The disease matter is in the system still—plus the drug poison.

After a time, when vitality has **sufficiently recuperated,** nature may make another attempt at purification; this time perhaps in another direction, but again her well-meant efforts are defeated. This process of suppression is repeated over and over again until the blood and tissues become so loaded with waste material and poisons that the healing forces of the organisms can no longer re-act against them by means of acute disorders, and then results—**the chronic condition,** which, in the vocabulary of the old school, is only another name for **"incurable."**

Now we are better prepared to understand the **modus operandi** of vaccination and its relationship to small pox. If vaccination actually prevents small pox, it can do so only in one way, and that is **by developing in the system smallpox in the chronic form of the disease.** From the explanation given above we know that "chronic disease" means that the system is so loaded with disease matter, and the vitality so low that the vital force is unable to rouse itself to acute eliminative effort. Having disease in the low, cold chronic form means that we are not able to have it in the acute form, but for reasons just given we should much prefer to have a disease in the acute forms and be rid of the morbid encumbrances in a few days or weeks than to be afflicted by the chronic form of the disease for years, or for a lifetime.

Small pox, like every other infectious disease, is a filth disease. It grows, as we shall see later on, in a scrofulous soil only, and the small pox eruptions mean "rapid elimination of scrofulous and tuberculous poisons from the system."

Therefore, if we have the choice, we should certainly prefer small pox to the vaccination. "Cheap talk," some one says. Not so, my friend, this is not merely talk—we were put to the test more than once in our own flesh and blood, and therefore we speak from experience and with authority.

© The Nature Cure Publishing Co., Chicago.

Naturopathy holds that germs, bacteria and parasites are products of disease rather than its cause.

When disease germs find in the human body the necessary conditions for growth and propagation— namely, lowered vitality, and their own congenial morbid soil—they multiply very rapidly and develop all the symptoms of that particular germ disease.

1911

Something Far-Reaching

J. T. Robinson, M.D.

———

Better Education

J. P. Bean, N.D.

———

Medical Persecution Of The Fasting Cure

Linda Burfield Hazzard, D.O.

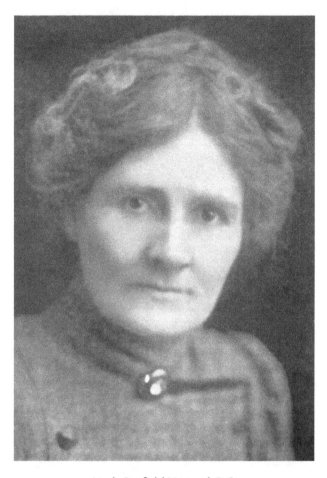

Linda Burfield Hazzard, D.O.
Fasting for the Cure of Disease, Physical Culture Corporation,
New York (1912).

Something Far-Reaching

by J.T. Robinson, M.D.

The Naturopath and Herald of Health, XVI(2), 106-107. (1911)

The American people should be forewarned, and forewarning is forearming.

Do they want an autocratic political bureaucratic medical trust as their dictator, with Theodore Roosevelt as the monarch of all that he surveys? Do you want your health and liberty regulated by an army of inspectors who are the agents and who are under the direction of this autocratic political bureau? Do you know that there are five bills before the present congress which, if passed, could be so used and the concealed purpose of which is to give supreme power to this trust?

Do you know that the terms of all the bills are so subtle that such bureau or department could at any time take action according to its interests or prejudice without specific legislation, and that the usual effect would be to commit the United States Government to the establishment of a system of old-time medicine, denying to the people the right to select for themselves the kind of medical treatment they shall employ? Do you know that William H. Welsh, as president of this gigantic, heartless, medical trust, has told the Senate Committee of Public Health and National Quarantine that the doctors wanted such a national department of health for the purpose of "influencing" the state and municipal boards of health? They are asking for supreme power to regulate and control health affairs nationally.

The American Medical Association has in the course of years developed into a political machine, simply for the purpose of bringing about legislation that will place it in absolute control of the nation's medical practice.

It is a war and the knife to the hilt between the old-time orthodox methods as against the great army of progress embracing all the new methods of the healing art throughout the entire world.

The question to decide is whether the intelligence of the twentieth century with all its advance and discovery be supplanted by the ignorance and superstition of the centuries that have passed.

In opposition to this mighty monster we have another organization known as the League for Medical Liberty, headed by B.O. Flower, of Boston, who founded the *Arena* magazine, and is now editor of the *Twentieth Century* magazine. Ex Governor John L. Bates, of Massachusetts, has been retained as principal counsel of the league, also Harry King, of Toledo, Ohio, is another distinguished lawyer who has been selected in the interest of the American people. Such legal lights will see to it that the medical trust will not outlaw all the new schools and thus become an engine of oppression. They will prevent the establishment of an autocracy and medical dictatorship.

Little did these old tyrannical medical leaders think of the mighty upheaval of public sentiment that was to confront them in the present Congress. Dr. Frank Lydston, of the medical faculty of Illinois State University of Chicago, is one of the insurgents of the American Medical Association. Charles W. Miller, member of the Iowa legislature, is vice-president of the League for Medical Freedom, and the A.P. Harsch, of Toledo, is the secretary. Many other brilliant men and women have joined this mighty movement together with the great masses of the American people, and will lay bare the dirty, designing, selfish schemes to rob, rule and murder millions of men, women and children all over the world.

These marauders and Tories as the enemies of our government have their agents in 900 counties in the United States. Any little two-by-four politician is the subservient tool of this heartless, robbing, murdering combination of cutthroats. The Standard Oil Company with its billions of ill-begotten wealth are humanitarians in comparison. These financial vipers may corner the markets of the world, but they do not lead millions of innocent women and children to the various slaughter pens to be butchered for mere pay. It is the weighing of money against life, the counting out of so many dollars against so many ounces of blood. Even now in the small town of Uvalde, Texas, the members of this political medical trust have had their fraudulent election contested.

The old sheriff who for more than twenty years has been holding office by fraud and deception, has a last been caught in his craftiness. The old political schemer has been successful in deceiving the people for a long time, but his nefarious plots have been unearthed, and he has recently been caught in the game of deception; he has sent out and had the unscrupulous and ignorant brought from adjoining counties and voted them illegally; he has defied investigation, law or order, but the old fox has been caught in his cunning; he is the veritable agent of the medical trust and political trust, and has been instrumental in arresting, fining and imprisoning the better element of physicians and laymen as a matter of graft, and because these people would not endorse his dark methods. These agents of the medical and political trusts have been found guilty of dark deeds in dark places among dark people. The agents of the political and medical grafters have been found guilty stuffing ballot boxes in as much as the transportation of ignorant Mexican and American voters from other countries, illegally cast may be termed stuffing. The old time dark chieftain, who for twenty years lived with the delusive impression that he had some mysterious divine right to rule the people of Malde County, now finds the people growing more intelligent to his disgust. The recent contest is an eye opener to the public. The people have reason to believe that this game has been played many times in the past of the wild and woolly West. The agents for the political and medical grafters will, no doubt, have to lick their calf over, and their more upright and honorable opponents will be at the licking. You can't fool the people all the time.

—San Antonio, Texas.

The American Medical Association has in the course of years developed into a political machine, simply for the purpose of bringing about legislation that will place it in absolute control of the nation's medical practice.

BETTER EDUCATION

by J.P. Bean, N.D.
The Naturopath and Herald of Health, XVI(3), 163. (1911)

Anent the attempts of the American Association to have laws in the different States practically prohibiting graduates of the irregular schools from practicing on the ground that they are ignorant, incompetent and a menace to public health, it is proper to remark that in a majority of cases they are dead right, though—truth to tell—if they are hunting quackery, incompetency and rascality, they had better begin by weeding out of their own ranks the "scrubs" and scoundrels who, under the protection of diplomas and licenses— obtained God knows how—are killing more people than get well in spite of their poisoning and slashing. No school or cult of healing could possibly turn out worse material than some of the "graduates" of some of the "regular" schools. In starting a movement for higher standards of education in the "regular" schools the American Medical Association is making a move in the right direction. But it is beyond question that the osteopathic and chiropractic, as well as the naturopathic schools are every year graduating some mighty poor material. They generally learn one thing pretty well, but do not learn enough of the essential accessory branches. This makes them exceedingly narrow and egotistical. The advertisements published by some of these people contain such a wealth of ignorance and conceit as to make excellent literature for the promoters of legislation to suppress frauds and quacks. An ignorant, conceited practitioner is a disgrace and an injury to the school from which he graduates. Now let us see what branches are essential to a good, practical medical education. (1) Anatomy and histology; in order that the student may know the size, location, shape and microscopic structure of the various organs. (2) Physiology, which treats of the functions of the organs. (3) Pathology, which treats of the morbid changes in structure and functions in disease of organs. (4) Diagnosis, which enables one to read and interpret the manifestations of disease. (5) General principles of therapeutics, especially those involved in his special line of work.

A thorough knowledge of these five branches lays a solid foundation of really scientific work. You must study these as long as you live —for you cannot learn them too well.

Now let us—as practitioners and students—each constitute himself a committee of one to raise the standard of naturopathic education and efficiency. Let us strengthen our weak points, improve our strong ones and by helping each other strive to lift our school to its rightful place. Your education at college is just a beginning of the higher, broader education that must be gained in the field of practical work. Study each patient and treat *him* and not the *disease*. It is well to be able to minister to a mind diseased, but you can do it better if you have a scientific knowledge of the structure and functions of the machine through which the mind works. The people are becoming better educated along the lines of health every year—thanks to the literature sent forth by the various new schools of healing. The medical practitioner of fifty years ago knew less of medicine than does the average layman of to-day. Practitioners of to-day must advance with the times or get out of the business. I don't think much of a man or institution that tries to sneak behind a bulwark of laws as a protection against honest competition. Real ability can always stand on its own merits. It is only incompetency that needs protection. Let us improve ourselves and at the same time teach our patients to know and appreciate merit. Then fallacy will die of itself.

Let us strengthen our weak points, improve our strong ones and by helping each other strive to lift our school to its rightful place.

MEDICAL PERSECUTION OF THE FASTING CURE

by Linda Burfield Hazzard, D.O.

The Naturopath and Herald of Health, XVI(12), 776-778. (1911)

Dr. Linda Burfield Hazzard of Seattle, Washington, has lately been arrested, charged with willfully starving one of her patients to death. Dr. Hazzard is widely known as a prominent advocate and practitioner of fasting for the cure of disease and has met with a large measure of success in her chosen field. She has been engaged in this work for the past fifteen years, and embarked upon it under the guidance of the late Dr. Edward Hooker Dewey. Like her preceptor she has been compelled to suffer malignment and persecution from the orthodox schools of medicine, and her career exhibits a history of continued effort on the part of the medical fraternity to ruin her practice and to decry her method.

Beginning her work in Minneapolis, when osteopathy was in its infancy, Dr. Hazzard now holds, in addition to her license as an osteopath, the only license in this country for the practice of fasting as a means of cure. The liberal law now on the statute books of the State of Washington that makes this possible and permits the recognition of the various methods of natural healing was passed by the legislature largely through her efforts, and she may well be considered as a shining example of what constant struggle against adverse conditions may succeed in accomplishing.

For the past five years Dr. Hazzard has been located in Seattle, Washington, and she has enjoyed a large and lucrative practice. So successful has she been that patients have sought her the world over. In all these years but twelve deaths have occurred under her care, and in each and every instance the post mortem examination revealed the cause as organic disease that made death inevitable fasting or feeding. The medical world through the public press and otherwise has assailed both physician and method whenever a death was announced, and her reiterated statements that structural and functional defects in the human body are largely the results of drugs administered in the developing period have called down upon her head the condemnation of orthodoxy to an extent hardly to be conceived.

In all ages, independence in thought and action, departure from orthodox methods, and the substitution of reason for superstition and tradition in the search for truth have called down protest, vituperation and persecution upon the individual or the sect that dared defy public opinion or established rule. The same acts that compelled the Puritans to emigrate from their native shores were in turn visited by them in severer form upon Roger Williams, Anne Hutchinson and the unfortunate Quakers.

The comparison of the treatment of disease in the human body by drugs with that through natural methods results in but one conclusion, and this is overwhelmingly in favor of nature's means of cure. The treatment of disease by drugs is purely an attempt to overcome the symptoms of disturbance. Medicine aims to stop or paralyze the signs of disease. Disease should be considered as a unity, arising from one cause, to be attacked at its source. The method indicated by nature strikes at its very roots; it removes the condition that causes the symptom. In all ways possible the natural method of treatment assists the organs of elimination to rid themselves of the products of the decomposition of excess food stored in body tissue, food ingested beyond the need for repair of broken-down cells. Medicine is at best but empirical in practice, an attempt to overcome symptoms by rule of thumb. "If at first you don't succeed, try, try again!" Barely more than a hundred years ago doses of "chamber tea," of dried powdered manure, and of spiders' legs were ordinary remedies. Washington was killed by the process of blood-letting, still common the latter half of the nineteenth century. And even the present generation remembers with disgust the close, drug-laden atmosphere of the fever room, where fresh air was prohibited, and water forbidden, while loathsome decoctions were forced upon the unwilling victim.

True, to-day these measures are abandoned, but the advocates of sunshine, pure air, water, and hygienic accessories were given the fight of their lives ere the light of truth penetrated this gloomy jungle of superstition and ignorance. In the world of medicine each departure from the customs of the past calls forth the ridicule and slander of the profession, and every advance in the progress of remedy and hygiene has been damned by the critics and their followers until its truth and its merit won recognition over scorn and determined opposition.

The medical fraternity visits its condemnation not only upon outsiders, but on those who have dared to differ within their own ranks. Reform in medicine has usually originated with the thinking lay mind. The profession has been forced in every instance to accept against its will the truth or its semblance. Witness the Pasteur treatment and the investigations later conducted upon the so-called germ theory.

This is the history of the introduction of vaccination into the curriculum of therapeutics, and this is now being seriously questioned by advanced thought; it was repeated again and again before the adoption of the germ theory, inoculation with serum, and all of the latter attempts at advance in hygienic care of the body and the community.

When Dr. Edward Hooker Dewey promulgated his advocacy of fasting for the cure of disease, he fully realized the seriousness of the struggle upon which he had entered. A graduate in medicine, he saw his colleagues turn upon him, repudiate his genius and his learning, and personally revile him. Often he tired of the fight and longed to lay his burden down, but the love of truth and of the message he bore to suffering humanity forbade relinquishing his pen and his practice until death brought release. He fought for his principle as founded on solid basis of truth, and he died a comparatively young man, a martyr to his cause.

For fourteen years the writer has advocated the theories that Dr. Dewey taught. They were not completely elaborated in their earlier form, but the experience of constant practice has brought them to the point of full understanding, and the application of nature's indicated means of rest for overworked human machinery through the abeyance of the digestive functions has won for itself a position in therapeutics that cannot be usurped nor overthrown.

In winning recognition the pathway has been strewn with obstacles that would have deterred a mind less forceful or a nature not convinced of the absolute truth and logic of its cause. Each step was taken against malignant and vicious persecution from sources least expected, but always traceable to the forces of organized medicine.

In five years past the fight has been waged in the State of Washington, where commercialism in the medical profession has so prostituted its honor that in fear of overproduction of licensed practitioners and of consequent distribution of fees, no college of medicine has been permitted the State University. Washington, where for similar reasons no license to practice medicine in another State is recognized, Washington, where a black-list of poor-pay patients exists, and, the Oath of Hippocrates to the contrary, no ailing body may be treated if the fee be not paid in advance.

The struggle has been long and difficult. It has led from the court of popular prejudice, the daily news, through police and superior courts, to the state legislature. And, won in the people's tribunal, it was forced to the supreme court of the state for interpretation. Garbled truths, falsehood, and vexations delay marked all the efforts to final successful issue; yet, though the privileges are granted, the struggle still goes on.

No stone has been left unturned by the medical world in order to find a pretext upon which to ruin me and my practice. In every case, the evidence introduced by the opposition had been expert medical evidence, and it was all naturally antagonistic to the cure, despite the proofs of post mortem examination. I may justly claim that I am the first investigator to call attention to the ravages of drug dosing in infancy. It is responsible for the larger portion of organic imperfections in the human body. Its effects are not so pronounced in adult life as in infancy, for the grown body has developed resistive powers not possessed by the child. Intestines of infantile size cannot be produced by the fast in a few days or weeks; gall stones to the number of 126 cannot be the product of 26 days of fasting; intussuscepted intestines of cartilaginous structure must have years to change from normal; and a cirrhosed liver takes as much time to alter in structure.

Each case of death cited came to only after medicine had done its worst, and each displayed organic imperfections that made death inevitable, fasting or feeding.

The two greatest crimes on earth are gossip and ignorance. The interference of officious neighbors and friends was responsible for the beginnings of each item of persecution related; their ignorance and that of the medical profession led to the active parts played by the medical world and the authorities. The ignorance that refuses investigation of a truth is harder to combat than that of a simple unlettered mind, and the regular physician is here exhibited as taking refuge in the fact that he is a graduate of some prominent school where such things as are advanced in fasting for the cure of disease were never taught, therefore they cannot be true, and must not be countenanced.

The injustice of the antagonism shown against this cause is exemplified in the fact that virtually all financial returns from a large practice have had to be devoted to the defense of the attacks made on me personally. Were it not that I am so fully convinced of the logic and truth of the method I advocate, and that I feel that I have proved beyond the shadow of a doubt that fasting is always a successful means for the restoration of health when organic disease is not present, I should have abandoned my work years ago. But in every death that has occurred under my care, a post mortem examination has invariably disclosed that death resulted not from the fast, but from some irremovable mechanical or structural defect in the body of the patient. And the successful cares are in number as the sands of the sea.

The medical world are now congratulating themselves that a cat's paw is at hand to push the case pending to a ruinous issue for both the cause and its advocates, but "He laughs best who laughs last," and the truth cannot be overcome. This article will have served its purpose if it but open the eyes and the minds of our readers to the necessity of independence of thought and of action in the search for truth, which is, after all, the only purpose of life on earth.

The editor will thankfully receive any amount in behalf of Dr. Linda Burfield Hazzard for the trial pending.

—Seattle, Wash., August 25, 1911.

1912

A Physical Culture History
Bernarr Macfadden

———

Naturopathic News
Benedict Lust

———

Friends Of Medical Freedom And Voters, Attention!
A. A. Erz, D.C.

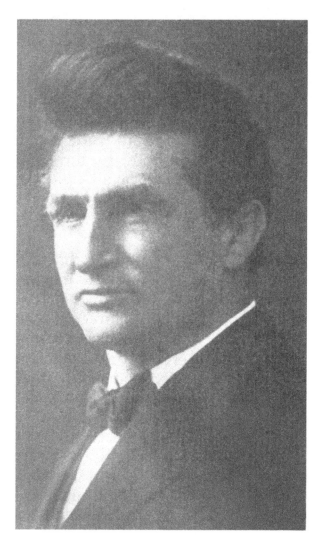

Bernarr Macfadden, N.D.

A Physical Culture History

by Bernarr Macfadden

The Naturopath and Herald of Health, XVII(1), 30-32. (1912)

From where the vast Atlantic beats against the Eastern shores of the Western Hemisphere to where the same great body of water is met by the Western coasts of European lands there are thousands of men, women, and children who believe in and practice Physical Culture: And of this mighty throng there are comparatively few who cannot tell something of the man who has done more than any other one person to spread the doctrine of health through intelligent exercise. And this man, Bernarr Macfadden, who instituted the *real* physical training which is gaining so many adherents each year was not always a physical culturist. Nor did he so much as dream of the wonderful part that he was to play in the great drama of life. Indeed had he done so he would probably have laughed to scorn the idea that his disease-stricken body would ever be strong and that the methods employed in attaining that strength would aid many more in the struggle for health with the resulting joy of living.

Adopted by a farmer in early life after the death of both parents, young Macfadden began a life of harsh treatment which continued until his twelfth year when he ran away. Drifting into St. Louis, Missouri, where he had relatives, he began working as an office boy and remained at office work until during his fifteenth year when his health which had undergone many vicissitudes, became so poor that he was compelled to desist. Every symptom was prophetic of a consumptive's grave, for not only was he weak, and emaciated, and afflicted with a hacking cough, but his mother had succumbed to that disease which was proof to the doctors and sympathetic friends that it was a case of heredity.

But young Macfadden was not one to give up without a strenuous effort to at least ameliorate his condition if it were not possible to effect a cure. He accordingly consulted doctor after doctor, and at the same time doped himself with patent drugs. But try as he would he did not only *not gain*, but rather lost. Driven by extremity he began to experiment with exercise with the idea that this might help him where other treatments had failed. From the first he made rapid improvement and realizing its wonderful curative qualities he continued the practice and at the same time extended his knowledge of different systems as they existed. The information thus gained combined with the interest which his own case aroused in him caused him to commence giving instruction along those lines. From St. Louis he went to New York, where he taught for some time, after which he spent several months in advertising an exerciser which he had invented. He later crossed to England and there he was accorded a more than casual attention by the masses of health seekers. Month after month passed and he still continued to grow in favor with those who crowded to hear him lecture. Recognizing the necessity of providing some better means of reaching the many whom he could not personally meet he established his first magazine. He still felt however that his best work lay in America and consequently he came back to New York City, where he secured desk room in a building on Broadway and started the publication of the *Physical Culture Magazine*. The business rapidly increased, compelling him to add office after office to accommodate the assistants whom he selected to help him, until at the time he moved to the present location of the magazine, he was occupying a suite of eight rooms, for which he was paying an enormous rental.

Shortly after moving to the new quarters he began experimenting with food stuffs with a view to furnishing nourishing food at low cost. In order to extend his experiments and to prove the truth of his beliefs he opened the first Physical Culture restaurant. However, it was not long until the crowds which flocked to the new institution necessitated the opening of others. After a time they were incorporated under the name, Physical Culture Restaurant Company. Since then they have extended their business to Boston, Philadelphia, Pittsburg, Chicago, and Buffalo in each city serving pure food: Nor have they reached their limit for now every prospect points favorably to the early occupation of many fields which the great western cities cause.

But publishing, teaching, and managing the Physical Culture restaurants was not enough to satisfy the rapacious appetite for work which was possessed by their promoter. He therefore planned a Physical Culture City from which all of the evils which menace the present day society were to be barred—a place that was to be a heaven for those who believed in the natural life. Purchasing a tract of some two thousand acres in New Jersey he opened it for settlement. From the first every prospect was flattering for its early colonization and especially was this true after the railroad erected a station-house. A post-office was partially promised and everything was moving toward the early culmination of the plans of their founder when the entire enterprise was thrown into confusion through the arrest of Mr. Macfadden, on the charge of sending obscene matter through the mails. This needed the probability of a post-office as well as started a long, hard struggle for justice, which was not secured until the matter was called to the attention of President Taft.

Up to the time of this occurrence Mr. Macfadden had done practically nothing in the way of using his knowledge in the cure of disease, having limited his efforts to building the "body beautiful." Nevertheless he was deeply impressed with its curative agencies and began extending his work along that line as soon as opportunity offered; later opening two sanitariums, one in England and the other in the United States, at Battle Creek, Michigan. He afterwards moved the latter to Chicago, where he continued to conduct it successfully until the past season, when he relinquished its management to others in order to lift some of the burdens from his shoulders. And even though he has done this he will still have more work than the average man, for he retains his editorship of *Physical Culture*, which is read by hundreds of thousands of intelligent people and through which he will continue to wage war on the "National Organization" to place in ascendency any medical school or cult; the compulsory vaccination law; and the numerous other conditions that are being pressed upon the people. His lecturing tours will be as extensive and he will also have his other interests such as the Physical Culture restaurants to engross his attention.

Nor would this sketch be complete without some mention for the extensive additions that Mr. Macfadden has made to health literature in the fifteen volumes of which he is the author. These works cover practically every phase of physical training as well as several works in a lighter vein. For some time he has been working on an encyclopedia of physical culture which promises to surpass his previous efforts. And when we realize that he is still comparatively a young man we may well watch with interest his future work, rightly expecting even more than he has so far accomplished. Especially may such results be looked for when it is recognized that his supporters are becoming more numerous every day, all of whom wish for him the best that the future holds.

> *Driven by extremity he began to experiment with exercise with the idea that this might help him where other treatments had failed.*
>
> *He was deeply impressed with its curative agencies and began extending his work along that line as soon as opportunity offered; later opening two sanitariums, one in England and the other in the United States, at Battle Creek, Michigan.*

Naturopathic News

by Benedict Lust

The Naturopath and Herald of Health, XVII(6), 389-393. (1912)

As the editor was away on an lecture tour, he was very busy with his big law suit and on the 24th met with an accident, broke his collar bone, so that he could not work or go around, he was practically unable to attend the different meetings of the Drugless Practitioners Societies in New York City; and as the secretaries of these societies failed to send in their reports as they should have done, we could not bring the regular news of the meetings.

A number of new arrests have been made recently. Naturopath Mautner, Mechanotherapist Page, Mechanotherapist Bromberg, Magnetopath Miltenberger, Chiropractor Duringer, and a half dozen other natural and drugless healers have been arrested and brought to court. Some of these cases have been tried, including the one of the editor and his assistant, and all lost. Others are under bail from $300 to $3,000, sitting in court every day until their case is called, are carried to the bench of justice like innocent lambs and fined money and prison sentences, as if they were the greatest criminals, enemies to mankind, foes to the welfare of society, scoffed at by the public, misrepresented and unfairly treated by the rotten press that is hired by this *Medical Trust*. The whole procedure in these law suits as seen in our courts to-day, reminds us of the time of the early Christian Era, where the Rome emperors and the rotten republic of Rome killed and murdered people by the thousands on account of their religious convictions.

During my law suit, I had to sit several days in court, and the cases that were tried brought forth such a corruption and immorality of society that you would believe that men like Naturopaths, who teach the people health, cleanliness, true morals, a higher and better life, should be looked up on by our government as benefactors and should be encouraged; but what do they receive? To look at the judges, as they sit in court, to look at these lawyers of the Medical Society, to look at the sleuths and emissaries and very doubtful characters of the employees of this *Medical Graft*, tells the whole story. To see day after day in the New York courts Mrs. Francisca Benecry going up on the witness stand, kissing the holy bible and sneering that she succeeded in trapping an innocent man or woman practicing natural methods, makes one ashamed of mankind in general and womanhood in particular. Such a woman as Mrs. Benecry I don't think has ever trodden the earth before. She swore on the witness stand that she called at my place, pretended fake paralysis of the leg, simulated a fainting fit, swore that she spoke to the editor on October 19th, when he can prove that he was not in New York City on that day. This gives us a look into the mirror of what kind of combination the Medical Society is made up of and what we are up against. Some of these emissaries of the Medical Society have been going around to Nature Cure institutions asking bribe and promising protection from the law. A former assistant lawyer of the Medical Society asked me how much money I would give him if he pulls me out, as he was in with the judge. Judging from this experience, the judges are also in with the Medical Society and very likely to get a large share of the fines collected from the Naturopath "criminals." The money that is collected from these fines minus the expenses of the court, goes to the Medical Society, and with this money they engage sleuths and detectives, who go around and work up cases. If there was no money in it, there would be no prosecution. If the Naturopaths all would go to jail, and no one would give bail, and no one would pay any fines, the Medical Society would stop all at once, and all the spitlickers and hell servants who are in the employ of this society would have to look for another job, that is, if they could get one.

Some of them are poorly dressed, have big holes in their shoes, and make the appearance of crooks at first sight. I would like to see what employer would engage them outside the Medical Society.

Now, the details of my law suit. Francisca Benecry claims to have called on October 16, 1911, at my institution, telling me that she had pains in her chest, and that she wanted to know whether the Nature

Cure would help her. This is lie No. 1. I remember distinctly, and also my stenographer testified to the fact that she said that she is, run down, lost her brother recently and has a lame leg. I told her if she wants to be treated for any ailment she would have to pass an examination first. She said she did not want any medical treatment, she simply wanted to try these baths and massage, and she wants to build up. She said on the witness stand that she asked me what N. D. means and I said that it means Naturopathic Doctor; as was proven by my own witness, I told her it means Naturopathic Director. I have never seen in my magazine or anywhere else in New York State, N. D. meaning something different. Of course the Medical Society sees danger everywhere. They are afraid of the letters N. D. Mrs. Benecry further testified that she took an electric light bath, was put in a tub after the electric light bath. She also said that the water had a peculiar color and a peculiar odor, very likely chemicals in it. Oh! Yes, chemicals, that's what they are after. She had a plain, simple electric light bath, and a wash down in Croton water, and as everybody knows, in October, on account of the frequent rains, the water had a peculiar color and the peculiar smell she testified about, we knew where that came from. Yes, there is a very bad odor about every sleuth of the Medical Society. She says she was wrapped up in porous sheets, covered with blankets. The nurse started pulling her toes, went up with the hands on her legs and over the spine, moved the legs up and down, pressed on the spine, moved the muscles, and heaven knows what else. As Mrs. Benecry has taken hundreds of treatments and got many massages, she ought to have known by this time that such procedure constitutes the application of massage. She certainly was not worthy of a good massage, but something else would have been the proper thing, but she is bound to get that someday, if she keeps up this infernal work. We don't need to take revenge in our own hand. The law of compensation will certainly not miss her.

In summing up the case, Judge Russel said that there is no evidence shown from either side that I or my assistant practised medicine, or that we held ourselves out as physicians, but under general law, under the paragraph of the amended law from September 10, 1910, we are guilty. Under that law it says that all material and mental means used for the restoration of health constitute medical practice, also that it is illegal to treat and advise. Now here you are. According to this, in New York City everybody is violating the medical law, especially anyone who does anything for health. Is it possible that our law makers could pass such a law? Was it really the intention of the legislature to put such a law before the people of the commonwealth of New York? I hardly believe it. To my understanding this law simply refers to the practice of medicine and surgery; neither of them we have practiced, as the court declared itself.

Judge Forker of Brooklyn, who was one of the three presiding judges, dissented and wanted us to go free, but the other two judges stuck together, and as they were the majority, so we were fined $100 each. The lawyer of the Medical Society, in making his final address to the court, pointing at me, said: "What this man, Mr. Lust, concerns, as he is well known in business, respected socially, as he has a high standing as editor of *The Naturopath*, a magazine for all these quack methods or drugless methods, as is known from one end of the country to the other, I would make a motion that in addition to a heavy fine of money, that you give him also a long prison sentence." What a nice compliment and what a great recognition of my work of eighteen years for introducing and upholding the Nature Cure.

I was commissioned in 1896 by the late Father Kneipp in Germany to go to America to introduce the Kneipp System. I was appointed by the German Nature Cure Society to establish branches here and to introduce the German Nature Cure in America. I received in 1899 from the Saxon government a medal and an honorary diploma for having succeeded in transferring the Kneipp and Nature Cure to the United States. I received great distinction and appreciation when I was at the different headquarters of our movement in Germany and England when I was over there five years ago, and here they point at me and brand me as a criminal. What is service to mankind and an educational work for the common good in Europe is a crime of the worst kind in New York City, in our free and democratic country.

Yes, my dear readers, it made me feel very bad standing there in a crowded court room and be branded as a criminal. This same mean, dirty society has carried me to the bar of justice over and over again for the last eighteen years, and now succeeded the first time in branding me as a criminal. This time they have done it. I know, my readers understand the situation and do not feel and think as these outcasts of mankind. The lawyer fees for these two cases cost me around $300, other expenses connected with it, and the $200 fine amount to over $500; but I herewith challenge the Medical Society, that they have accomplished nothing, each dollar, also the other $1,000 which I have spent previously for lawyer fees to defend myself, will mean a new pioneer for natural methods. I will see to it, and I am going to work for co-operation and financial assistance to get a college established *right here in the city of New York for drugless methods, for the NATURE CURE,* that includes all that is good in the healing art, a college that is broad enough to include all good agents for the restoration and maintenance of health. It will be a school of health, preventive medicine, and no superstitious, old, worn out guess work of medical dummies.

It has come to pass that medicine stands to-day for intolerance, that this MEDICAL TRUST has acquired power over life and death, is in a position in New York to shut out every system of healing, every physical and mental help, except the three schools which have been recognized, besides themselves. That is the Eclectic, the Homeopaths and the Osteopaths. I want to say right here that behind this Medical Trust in New York State are to a large extent also the Osteopaths. Who are these Osteopaths? They are men who stood together in New York State, put up the money and after years of battering with the Medical Trust, the door was finally opened and they were let in. The majority of those who were let in at that time were men of no elementary education to speak of. They were nine week, five month and nine month Osteopaths, who happened to have seen the city of Kirksville when it was yet very easy to get a diploma as Osteopath. What is Osteopathy? It is nothing new. It was practiced and known, of course not under the name of Osteopathy, for centuries in Japan, China, Bohemia, England,

Germany, Denmark, and Sweden. Dr. Still certainly has added to it, and discovered some of these movements, but is Osteopathy as such a real system of healing? Does it cover all cases and conditions? It was not very long ago that they taught in Kirksville at their school and in their textbooks that it is not necessary to pay any attention to diet, habits and general hygiene. That Osteopathy is a cure all. Who would accept such nonsense to-day? Now, this hand full of Osteopaths in New York City have all worked hand in hand with their sleuths and the emissaries of the Medical Society to go around and to get evidence that Osteopathic movements were used by other practitioners than regular Osteopaths. Up in the State some have been arrested and fined. Now, what does all this mean? It simply means that we have class legislation pure and simple in New York State, and that all Allopaths, at least the largest majority of them who belong to-day to the Medical Trust, want to control the healing art, and want to shut out and close the door for every new system or help that has come up or may yet come up to relieve and cure human ailments. If anybody has a new discovery to-day that cures and relieves sickness and suffering, he cannot bring it forth in New York State. He would be arrested and branded as a criminal first, his ambitions and enthusiasms killed in him and he would have to throw off the dust from his feet and get out of New York.

Last week Congressman Work of California said in the Congress at Washington, when the discussion came up about this new department of health, and the unjust persecutions of the Christian Scientists in New York City, that if Jesus Christ himself would come to New York to-day, he would be locked up in 24 hours as a criminal for healing the sick. According to the law as it stands on the statute books, all material and mental means for the restoration of health constitutes medical practice. According to that, praying to the Lord for health is also a misdemeanor, and if the doctors were not afraid of the power of the different religious denominations, they would arrest every minister and every person who goes to church. If they were not afraid of the public's opinion they would arrest every proprietor of the Turkish baths, gymnasium, barber shops, hairdressers, chiropodists, in fact anyone who dares to give a bath or rub the head or touches or cleanses the body, as according to law and its present interpretations they have a perfect right to do so.

Mrs. Francisca Benecry said on the witness stand that she visited my institute over and over again. Yes, I remember very well when she came in at my place on the 59th Street one morning and told me that she had shooting pains in her chest and if I would not be so kind and give her something for momentary relief. I knew who she was, I knew her very well at the time. What did she do, she stood up from the chair and fell backwards down on the carpet and moaned and pretended a hysterical fit. I raised her up from the floor and turned her out to the door and told her that Dr. Kelley's office is right across the street. Yes, Mrs. Benecry has been trying for eight years continuously to get evidence against my institution. She even said on the witness stand that she was looking up my institution at one time for "something else"? Must be a terrible place a Nature Cure institute, according to Mrs. Benecry. When she came in October she wore a heavy veil. She was so dressed up that nobody could see her face, but I knew she was a detective and I told the nurse to give her a bath and massage, as I did not think anybody in the world could make out of a bath and massage treatment a violation of the medical law.

Other sleuths, men and women have visited my institution regularly. One day a man came in. He looked as if he was out of a job and when I came to the parlor he pulled out of his vest pocket a sputum receptacle and held it right up against my nose, asking me whether he had consumption or not. I got mad, of course I knew this dirty creature is another emissary of the Medical Graft, and I threw him out.

In November, 1904, just after I returned from a trip to Florida, I was told by my assistant and my wife that while I was away, day after day detectives came in inquiring for Dr. Lust. They were told that I would be back on such and such a day. I came home at eleven o'clock in the morning, at twelve o'clock there were already two women detectives in the parlor, one waiting for some treatment, and the other one wanted some remedy. I knew who they were and I chased them. The next morning at eleven o'clock I was sitting in my editorial office dictating letters, when a man came in and asked me if I was Dr. Lust. I said I am Mr. Lust, and told him to sit down until I finished dictating my letter, and when I turned and looked at him, he held up his two hands and then rubbed his two knees and said: "I have syphilis in my hands and knees and I want to try your cure." At the same moment, a second man came in and asked me if I am Mr. Lust. I said yes, and he handed me a warrant of arrest on which it said that party so and so against B. Lust for practicing medicine and surgery without a license. I read the paper and then he gave me the second one. On this one it said, the people of New York State against B. Lust for practicing surgery without a license. When I was brought to court, the first man who called, and whose name was on the first warrant, was an assistant lawyer of the Medical Society. I had never seen the man before, I had spoken nothing to him than to sit down, and there you see the warrants had been issued before he called at my place. That's how the law is handled in New York, that's the rights and protection dished out to citizens and taxpayers. On the way to court, this dirty lawyer of the Medical Infernal Machine, after he sent the detective away, asked me on the corner of 59th Street and Lexington Ave. to go with him in a saloon and that he would talk this affair over with me, and as he is in with the judge, he would settle the whole matter. Next he asked me how much money I have? That the whole machine was corrupt I could see at once. Now, if this society can have warrants issued and can have them counteracted by their lawyers, and can send the detective away with the warrant, that shows there is something wrong and there does exist a corrupt connection between the Medical Society and the judges. I told that grafty lawyer that I am not afraid of him, that I am not a criminal and that I am perfectly able to take care of myself and to face these charges. When I came to court I had sufficient evidence that that man was really "in with the judge." He would give me no chance to explain matters and simply said that he is no authority to decide whether Nature Cure is a violation of the medical law and he put me under $600 bail and asked me if have a bondman and a lawyer.

I am not through yet with the Medical Society. They glorify themselves in New York newspapers lately that they got all the graduates of my school arrested, about twenty-one of them, and they will see that my school and my institution will be closed. Nothing of the kind. I am here yet. I am yet at the old stand on Lexington Avenue, and the Medical Society has got the best for a while, but our turn will come for sure. The people of the State of New York will be shaken up. They will be informed what this medical combination is doing, and we will do it. I am preparing at present a little booklet that will expose one hundred cases of malpractice of regular medical doctors, a good many of them members of this autocratic, narrow-minded Medical Society. I want to mention just one case, which is just at present at our Health Home YUNGBORN, Butler, N. J. A young man of twenty years went to a doctor, asking him about some sexual disorder. The doctor advised him to visit a house of shame once a week. The young man was ashamed at such advice and said to the doctor, "Why, I may get some disease." The doctor replied, "Well, if you should catch something, I will treat you." This young man followed this doctor's advice and really got something, and the doctor treated him. To-day he has syphilis in the worst degree and his mind has given away and if it were not for the NATURE CURE, with which we can do something for this poor man, he would be a lost case.

Now this one case shows what the doctors are doing. These men who get laws on the statute books in the different legislatures to safe-guard the welfare and health of the people are the only ones who, for the sake of the greedy dollars, wreck lives and mutilate the innocent, and then they are considered benefactors and protectors of mankind.

At a recent banquet in New York City, Prof. Robinson said, to license Naturopaths and other drugless practitioners would simply mean to license the practice of crime. The fact really is, that M.D. to-day, the way it looks, is really a license for crime. He said the truth, but we have to reverse it and apply it to them. Do Naturopaths poison the blood of the people? Do they sacrifice healthy children to this demon of medical cursedness? Do they perform unnecessary operations? Do they teach nonsense in the teaching of health? The fact is that naturopaths and other drugless practitioners are the only ones who treat in conformity to the laws of Nature, remove the causes, establish cleanliness where there is dirt and disease, and regenerate the human body and teach the people the laws of preservation and restoration of health. The M.D.'s do just the contrary, they only treat symptoms all the time, they never remove the cause, they never tell the people anything about the prevention of disease. A Naturopath is a teacher of the common people. He is a sincere and honest man, in fact he sacrifices himself for the interest of his fellowmen and shows the people how to get along without any treatment at all. We have hundreds and thousands of such Samaritans and good physicians and doctors who take the whole man or woman into consideration, the mind and the body, and treat them with love and sympathy and help them.

I have been practicing as a Naturopath for eighteen years. Thousands of men and women have come to my two institutions. They were treated with Nature Cure methods and restored to health. They have learned how to live, how to take care of themselves, and they are grateful. Who were these people in most cases? They were patients who had made the whole round of doctors and specialists, who robbed them and who wrecked them physically and financially. When they had no more money the doctors gave them up, could not do anything for them. These greedy doctors for fifty years have been fighting amongst themselves what medicine really is. They can never give a proper definition anyway, but they succeeded in New York to include everything under the sun, God's own sun rays, the light and the water, the exercise, and the rest, even your prayer to the Lord, it's all medicine. It was only a short while ago that all drugless methods were quack methods; now they say it is all medicine. They opposed as long as they could. When they saw that the people found out that there is some good in it, now it belongs to them. There you are, in the year 1905, when I was up for trial at the Court of Special Sessions and I won my case, my lawyer introduced me after the trial to the lawyer of the Medical Society. He said, "I introduce to you Mr. Lust; he is not such a bad man as you think." The lawyer said, "Indeed, I think Mr. Lust is sincere and a perfect gentleman, but it is that "KNEIPP CURE", which he stands for, we are up against."

Champ Andrews, formerly chief lawyer of the Medical Society, said on a Sunday afternoon at the Y.M.C.A. on 57th Street, where he gave an illustrated lecture of quacks and quack methods: "After my ten years' connection and as chief lawyer of the Medical Society, I found out that the real quacks are the doctors themselves, and that all the different quacks and practitioners of irregular schools do not do much harm as the regular doctors." He said that after he was not in the services any more of this MEDICAL TRUST.

Yes, dear people of New York State, according to the present law, anything which prevents disease or sickness is medical practice and you cannot even have your corns attended to, neither can you take a health bath, or take a physical culture, or apply electricity or magnetism, you cannot engage in special breathing; in fact, you are not allowed to take a deep breath anymore without violating the laws of your State. If it is a crime for a Naturopath to apply the agencies of Nature, to help you and to heal you, then it is also a crime for you to take them.

What I have written here, I have said in good faith, and I am ready to prove it; if the medical doctors want to arrest me, all right, they are welcome. I will not run away.

A Naturopath is a teacher of the common people. He is a sincere and honest man, in fact he sacrifices himself for the interest of his fellowmen and shows the people how to get along without any treatment at all. We have hundreds and thousands of such Samaritans and good physicians and doctors who take the whole man or woman into consideration, the mind and the body, and treat them with love and sympathy and help them.

Friends Of Medical Freedom And Voters, Attention!

by A. A. Erz, D.C.
The Naturopath and Herald of Health, XVII(11), 707-709. (1912)

All intelligent, progressive readers are fully aware of the fact that one of the greatest needs of our time is *medical freedom,* and that the present medical laws of most States are far from being just and fair, and greatly in need of revision to do justice to the people. Yes, people are awakening, and the spirit of justice, liberty, and progression is still alive in this great country of ours. We all realize that something has to be done to change existing wrong conditions. Legislation is one means to change matters to some extent. In order to start properly, we will have to see to it that we have the right kind of law-makers in our legislatures. At this point the responsibility of every citizen and voter comes in and urges him to do his duty.

You, the voters of every State in the Union; you, the worth-while citizens of every town and city of the United States, must do your solemn duty on every election day, if you want to enjoy your liberty and individual freedom. The voting power is one of the greatest forces in the civilized world today, by which we can bring changes about for the good of all. By voting for the right man in the right place, we help sustain the constructive principle in operation in our laws and courts.

Our present medical laws are a mere farce as far as medical freedom and protection of the people are concerned; they are framed up by the political doctors to humbug the public and to perpetuate the control of the antiquated medical system. These doctors represent a shrewdly organized, powerful trust that reaches out over every State, and makes itself felt everywhere through its County, State and National societies, in the strenuous effort to exercise all possible influence, and to secure patronage and power. They have a controlling influence in almost every newspaper. By their position they are in link with the money forces, the commercial and social interests, and party politics. It is a standing order of the American Medical Association to see to it that they are well represented in all movements and watch for a chance to manage matters in their own interest. At the present time, they are especially active in politics, and are trying to capture as many public offices as possible. The declaration of medical tyranny contained in our medical laws has been originated and indorsed by the medical trust of the political doctors known as the A. M. A. To do away with obnoxious medical legislation is to have the old laws abolished and proper new laws enacted for the proper protection of the rights of the people and the progress of the science and art of healing. The policy of all medical legislation in the past has been to force the mandates and tyranny of the old medical school upon the people. History shows that such course has ever been the last resort of an oligarchic class to remain in power and make everybody obey its mandates. The political doctors always refer to the letter of the *law*. Not justice and right, but the *law* must be observed! The medical law which has been arranged by the medical trust and enacted for the benefit of the medical doctors, is but class-legislation, pure and simple. The supposed protection of the people, about which the medical hypocrites have so much to tell you, is mere show and pretence to deceive the legislators and to soothe the people.

In medical laws of this kind no thought is given to the welfare of the people or to their conditional and God-given rights. Their real object is to keep out competition and to prosecute the drugless healer. True progress and advancement in the science and art of healing are thus made impossible by such paternalistic legislation asking protection for antiquated methods and dangerous practices. Medical laws stand for fencing in of the healing profession for one school only. Thus every citizen is denied the right to select the physician of his own choice, and patronize the school of his conviction.

It is not sufficient to protest against the enactment of any of the numerous restrictive medical measures which have been urged by the political doctors in every State of the Union. It is far better to do all in our power to prevent all such unfair legislation, and to have the present unjust medical laws repealed or properly amended. If you want to preserve your rights under the Constitution you will have to fight medical monopoly and graft by voting for such candidates only who are for medical freedom, in order to get reliable representatives into our legislatures, both State and Federal.

Every candidate for a legislative body, be it Federal, State or municipal, must state how he stands on the question of medical freedom before he can expect to get our vote. Remember that we have just the kind of laws we are deserving, and that it is our fault when our medical laws are a disgrace to a liberty loving people. Because we fail to do our duty on election day, and we send men to our legislatures not qualified to perform the act of law-makers of a generous, free, and democratic republic.

Voters should be careful whom they support for legislative positions and for city, town and county councils, demanding pledges of the candidates that they will never be parties to the enactment of laws which infringe the rights of all for the benefit of the few. Let every reader attend to his duty as a citizen at the voting box, and by urging his friends to support only those candidates for office who are friends of medical freedom.

It takes men of ripe education and knowledge of the world, wise in experience and action, conscientious and liberal in their dealings with mankind, to make good laws for the betterment of humanity, and to execute them. It is high time that the people in general are getting a truly representative government. Political evolution treads slowly, but progress moves always toward the light, justice, and the square deal. If at times it records seeming recession, it comes all the stronger in its later strides and registers great in the pages of history.

While the medical subjugation has gradually come about the entrenched political doctors have held high their heads in defiance of the rights of citizens, and imposed their tyranny upon the people. But their doom is bound to come. Continued discussion of the question of medical freedom has quickened the public conscience to a sense of right and wrong, and people are up in arms against inconsiderate, unfair, and tyrannical methods of the doctors. It is a struggle of great forces, and victory is sure to come to the friends of justice and liberty.

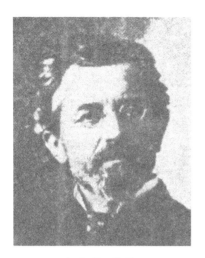

A. A. Erz, D.C.

The political doctors backed by the money power of the drug business, are just now very active in the political field. The order has been given by the A. M. A. to "pack" the Legislatures and Congress, in order to secure all the laws needed for the realization of their far-reaching political schemes. It is up to the voters to put a halt to all that and protect the rights and liberties of every citizen, woman and child.

The average voter keeps voting all his voting life without paying much attention to the personal standpoint on medical laws taken by the candidates for legislative offices for whom he is voting. Yet it is the duty of every voter to know how each candidate for legislature stands on so vital a question as medical freedom, in order to obtain the right kind of law for the benefit of all. Otherwise our legislatures will be "packed' with political doctors and their friends, and the laws they are making will be for their own benefit.

Every voter must see to it that the political doctor is kept out of the law making business and made to remain at home in his office where he belongs. A true physician is not supposed to spend his valuable time in politics, but to devote himself to the duties of his calling. A competent doctor should be able to acquire a practice which will pay better than any public office of the school board city council, or health departments pays. Those who take such jobs do it because they cannot earn a living legitimately, and they want to keep the medical trust in control of public offices for the benefit of themselves. The attitude of the political doctor in any public office is too selfish and malicious as far as medical freedom is concerned; his mind is out of step with progress and out of sympathy with the welfare of the people. His only aim is to help perpetuate medical despotism and to crush out all other systems of healing. And such a man is not in spirit with you as a proper representative of a progressive, liberty loving citizen.

It is the sacred duty of every voter to see to it that men get into office who have a heart that beats right and true with that side of humanity that works for the uplifting of all, and for the protecting and sustaining against such combinations of oppression and influences that are opposed to the square deal of man to man. Let us vote for such men only who believe in equity, justice, and freedom to all alike, and in privileges to none. ("Eternal vigilance is the price of liberty.") San Francisco

> *Their real object is to keep out competition and to prosecute the drugless healer.*
>
> *The order has been given by the A. M. A. to "pack" the Legislatures and Congress, in order to secure all the laws needed for the realization of their far-reaching political schemes.*

1913

DR. B. LUST'S RECREATION RESORT
"YUNGBORN"
BUTLER, N. J.
IN THE RAMAPO MOUNTAINS

Natural Life and Rational Cure Health Home for Dietetic-Physical-Atmospheric Regeneration Treatment. Fount of Youth, and New Life School for those in need of Cure and Rest, for the physically and spiritually weakened, for those overworked and for the convalescent.

OPEN ALL THE YEAR

Winter Branch: *Florida Yungborn, Tangerine, Florida*

IN the vicinity of the beautiful country town of Butler, N. J., there spreads, in incomparably ideal beauty, surrounded by majestic pine forests, orchards and parks, the Health Resort of YUNGBORN. The establishment was called a *Yungborn* by reason of the rejuvenating and strength-endowing effects of its Regeneration Cures. And indeed, these extensively known Yungborn-Regeneration Cures are not only health-restoring, but also Rejuvenating and Strength-giving Cures. Already during, and particularly after the treatments are completed, the strength and vitality, formerly low and broken, rise with astonishing assurance. Vital energy and vital strength return; increased nerve-elasticity and an undreamed-of sensation of powerful health make themselves felt. And with the new creative power there asserts iself a feeling of spiritual and physical rejuvenation and unlimited efficiency.

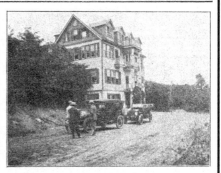

Yungborn Regeneration Cures—
The dietetical Regeneration Cures which are applied in their particular gradations as required for the various diseases and conditions of weakness, are fully adapted to the case in hand and modified correspondingly.

The most peculiar and most intense forms of these Cures are the *Schroth Treatment*, so called after its founder, the genial Johann Schroth, and the combined *Diet, Light-Air and Water Treatments* in which the experiences of *Schroth, Kneipp, Rickli, Lahmann, Ehret, Just, Engelhardt*, etc., are resorted to individually. Furthermore, Fruit Cures, Herb Cures, Vegetal and Mixed Diet, Fasting Diet Cures in combination with Fruit Diets, and so forth. Diet requires individually adapted physical treatment, such as *packings*, bandaging, baths and gushes of various descriptions, barefoot walking, light, *sun* and *air baths*, steam, electricity, massaging, Osteopathy, Chiropractic, Mechanotherapy, Neuropathy, etc. Special attention is given to the development of humid warmth treatment as one of the most important curative factors.

Aid in Obsolete, Inveterate Cases—
The Yungborn Regeneration Cures will help even in the most deep-rooted and superannuated sufferings and conditions of weakness, where other cures failed, except in cases of organic new growth and destructions (like cancer and consumption) or marasmus.

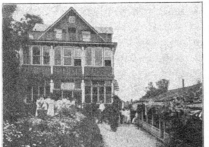

It need hardly be mentioned that not only those requiring cure, but also those *in need of rest*, the weakened and convalescing derive the best possible benefits of lasting effect from a sojourn at the Yungborn.

Fall, Spring and Winter Cures—
We wish to call the reader's attention particularly to the fact that the *Yungborn is also splendidly suited for a stay in winter time.* Not only the Regeneration but also the Strengthening Cures are immensely successful in winter. In addition, the delightful, mild *forest and mountain air* so rich in ozone and oxygen, is of extraordinarily vivifying, refreshing and strengthening effect upon the entire organism (which is true of every season).

Dr. B. Lust's Recreation Resort "Yungborg" Butler, N.J.

Benedict Lust's Health Resorts:

"Yungborn," Butler, N.J., and "Qui-si-sana," Tangerine, Fla.

by Benedict Lust

The Naturopath and Herald of Health, XVIII(7), 496-500. (1913)

Location

Benedict Lust's Health Resort "Yungborn" is located near Butler, N. J., a picturesque and prosperous little country town of some four thousand inhabitants. This part of New Jersey is known as the Ramapo Mountains and renowned for its pure, invigorating air, its scenic beauty and its numerous mountain lakes.

Butler, N.J., is only one hour's ride from New York on the Susquehanna and Western Branch of the Erie Railroad and also easily accessible by automobiles from all directions.

This is one of the reasons why the institution is so well patronized by New Yorkers as a vacation resort and a convenient place for week-end trips.

Environment

The state of a patient's mind is of great importance in the treatment of disease. There is no greater obstacle to the progress of recovery than worry, and no more powerful aid than a cheerful disposition.

It, therefore, is the policy to make the patient's surroundings as pleasant as possible and, by eliminating everything that is suggestive of a hospital, cultivate a health-inspiring spirit which is bound to greatly increase the effectiveness of the treatment.

Method Of Treatment

Any real and permanent cure must be the result of a change in the body itself. There must be a constitutional reconstruction which can be brought about only by the operation of the great forces of Nature, which are concerned in the development and maintenance of all living beings.

There is no artificial treatment which embodies these principles. Every artificial treatment is more or less symptomatic and as such admissible in incurable diseases where the object of the treatment is to ease the patient's suffering, and occasionally in temporary afflictions in which the symptoms require immediate relief, while a speedy removal of their cause is impossible.

However, to treat an established curable disease merely symptomatically, as a great many patients are inclined to do, is decidedly wrong. Symptoms are but the manifestation of the disease, not the disease itself, and to direct our efforts towards them, instead of their cause, is like chopping off the leaves of a weed to kill the plant.

We can suppress most any symptom by means of a remedy, we can produce sleep in a person suffering from chronic insomnia by dose of veronal, we can relieve chronic headaches by administering aspirin, we can cause an evacuation of the bowels in chronic constipation by a laxative, we can suppress the symptoms of chronic rheumatism by administering salicylates, we can quiet a neurasthenic by sedatives, we can lessen the frequency of convulsions in an epileptic by bromides. But we do not cure in this manner.

If we discontinue the treatment, the former symptoms, as a rule, will reappear, and if we continue it, we may do the patient irreparable harm.

In order to cure a disease, it must be our object to abstain from sympathetic treatment as much as possible and engage the entire cell action in the repair work which has to be done, instead of burdening it with additional work which is incurred in the process of eliminating the drug.

The power that cures a disease lies in the patient himself. It is called the Vis Medicatrix Naturae, i.e., the inborn healing power which exists in every living body. It is the dominant force which in sickness as well as in health moves and regulates the circulation of the blood, the action of the lungs, the processes of digestion and assimilation, the function of the kidneys, muscles, nerves and every other organ of the body.

To act upon and strengthen this natural healing power is the object of the method of treatment employed at this institution. The means by which we try to accomplish this purpose are the following:

Outdoor life, sun and air baths, diet, water treatment, systematic exercises, massage, rest cure.

As simple as these treatments seem, they are most powerful if scientifically applied, i. e., applied in conformity with the requirements of each individual case.

OUTDOOR LIFE

There is nothing more injurious to health than breathing impure air. To spend most of our time, as the majority of us do, in stuffy offices, stores or shops, and in overheated and poorly ventilated living and sleeping rooms is against the very first principle of health culture and will, in the course of time, lead to disastrous results.

Headaches, irritability, a defective digestion, sluggish bowels, an anemic and a general feeling of mental and physical lassitude or weakness are, as a rule, the first signs of a failing health.

Breathing pure air is the first essential for the preservation of health and is, consequently, particularly important for the restoration of health.

There is no virtue in any method of treatment which disregards this fundamental law of Nature.

Without pure air there is no healthy blood, and without healthy blood there is no cure. It matters little what the character of the affliction. The cure of a skin disease, for instance, depends upon a healthy condition of the blood, the same as the cure of consumption.

Trying to cure a complicated chronic disease without the aid of outdoor life is a futile effort and a waste of time.

In constructing the sleeping cottages it has been our aim to provide the most perfect ventilation and thus enable the patient to breathe pure country air every minute of his stay at the institution, day and night.

SUN BATHS

Sunlight is as essential for the welfare of a human being as it is for a living plant. It is the most powerful force in Nature, without which there is no healthy or natural development.

You may try the experiment in your garden. Plant two flowers of the same species, age and size, but in different locations, one where it gets the sunshine all day long, and the other where it is shaded part of the day. Provide the two plants with the same rich soil and take equally good care of both. Then study their further growth. One will sprout into a healthy plant, while the other will show but a poor growth and never equal the splendid development of the other.

The same applies to the human body. The one who lives in the light of the sun will develop a healthy mind and body, while the one who is condemned to a sedentary life will wither and soon begin to show the signs of disease and premature age.

The action of the sunlight increases the activity of every organ and every cell, and the more perfectly and harmoniously these perform their functions the healthier we are.

Of particular importance is the action of sunlight upon the activity of the skin, the function of which as an eliminative organ is as essential as that of the kidneys. Through its millions of pores it removes part of the impurities which constantly accumulate in the system and often cause a condition of the blood which is called toxemia or auto-intoxication (self-poisoning).

To stimulate the elimination of these various poisons which are the cause of many constitutional diseases, such as rheumatism, gout, neurasthenia, etc., is one of the purposes of judiciously applied sun baths.

The sun baths at this institution are not given under a glass roof, which consumes the most important rays of the sunlight, but in the open. Two secluded enclosures one for women and one for men, provide absolute privacy, and the patient is at liberty to enjoy the full benefit of an ideal sun and air bath.

DIET

The purpose of food is to provide those elements which are required to reconstruct the material which has been consumed by the various activities of the body. Every thought, every muscular contraction, every heart-beat, in short every physical and mental effort, consumes certain elements which are to be replaced.

Considering our absolute lack of knowledge as regards the mysteries of metabolism, it is impossible to prescribe with any degree of exactness the proper diet in any one particular disease.

Individualizing, i. e., to adapt the diet to the individual patient and not so much to the character of the disease, is the secret of dietetics.

There are no two individuals alike, and the fact that two patients are afflicted with the same disease does not justify a physician in providing both with the same food elements. What is meat for one may be poison for the other.

In conformity with this principle, we do not insist on any particular diet, but serve a mixed, vegetarian, milk, raw food, and any other special diet as each individual case may require.

Under certain conditions we advise a systematic fast, provided the patient possesses the necessary vitality.

WATER TREATMENTS

The water cure (hydrotherapy) has been employed in an empirical way since ancient times. To-day it is an established scientific method which is advocated and practiced by every progressive physician and taught in every modern Naturopathic school. To-day we not only know that certain applications of water have certain effects, but we also know why they have these effects. We know that properly applied water treatments regulate or modify the circulation of the blood, deepen the respiration, increase the number of blood cells, assist the elimination of toxins through the kidneys and skin, in short improve the activity of every organ and cell of the body.

Water treatments, if properly applied, are the most powerful means to build up and invigorate a nervous weakened system and enliven a tardy digestion and assimilation.

Owing to its flexibility, the water cure can be applied to every constitution, strong or feeble.

EXERCISES

Regular exercise is as important for the preservation and restoration of health as breathing pure air and eating proper food. It brings into play every part of the organism, improves the activity of every organ. It teaches coordination of mind and body, will power and self-control.

It stimulates physical and mental vigor, restores and strengthens self-confidence, creates anew the love of living and doing and keeps us from growing old. Continuous activity physical and intellectual is the chief preventative of old age.

"It adds years to our life and life to our years." Lack of activity, on the other hand, causes a sluggish circulation, weak lungs and poor digestion, and thus leads on to misery and premature age.

The physical exercises at the institution are given in the air-bath, where the patients are not hampered by uncomfortable clothing, and are graduated according to the character and stage of the disease and the physical strength of the patient. Apart of these exercises are ample opportunities for all kinds of outdoor sports and games, swimming and cross-country walks. The patients also have an opportunity to assist in gardening and at farming, if they so desire.

Special exercises, so-called orthopedics, are given to children being afflicted with deformities. By combining these exercises with an outdoor life and other natural methods very successful results are obtained.

MASSAGE

Massage treatments are particularly beneficial in feeble and nervous patients whose lack of vitality disables them to participate in active physical exercises.

Massage, particularly if combined with so-called Swedish movements, is one of the most effective means to improve the circulation of the blood and a sluggish lymphatic flow, to stimulate weak muscular tissues, to maintain and increase suppleness by stretching ligamentous structures and to strengthen the nervous system.

Locally applied, it is a splendid help in numerous localized diseases. In chronic constipation, for instance, there is no more effective treatment than abdominal massage, in combination with certain kinds of exercises and water applications.

Rest Cure

Rest does not mean simply eating and sleeping. Rest, in the first place, consists in a relief from the monotony of our daily life, i.e., a change of occupation and surroundings or environments.

A person who overworked himself in one direction will find the proper test in converting his activities into entirely different channels. Some outdoor game, a walk through the woods or country, a little work in the garden will furnish the proper rest for the exhausted professional or business man, while the one who overworked himself physically will find the necessary rest by spending his time "in dolce far niente," or in some light outdoor occupation.

How or to what extent the patient shall exercise or rest depends entirely upon his individual condition.

No set rule applies to any case. Occasionally it is advisable to keep the patient in bed for some time and limit the treatment to general and local massage, various packs and water applications, etc., all depending, of course, upon the condition of the patient.

How To Live

The object of the institution is not merely to cure those who are sick, but at the same time teach them the science of health culture.

If the patient does not learn how to take care of his health in the future, and he continues his former mode of living, he cannot expect the cure to remain permanent and absolute.

The same cause, the same result. To instruct him in all matters pertaining to health and disease is the object of popular lectures which are held one evening of each week.

How Much Time Does A Rest Cure Require?

This is a question often asked. The time required to perfect a cure varies considerably in all cases. Everything depends upon the character and obstinacy of the disease and the vitality and recuperating power of the patient.

It is unreasonable to expect something that is impossible and not give Nature a chance to do her work.

A disease which has existed for years cannot be cured within a few weeks.

A patient with a low vitality cannot expect to be cured as quickly as a more vigorous person.

Success, like in everything else, depends upon perseverance.

Many a patient could have been cured had he not expected the impossible and become discouraged because he did not see immediate results.

THE INSTITUTION AS A VACATION RESORT

There are two ways to spend a vacation. One way is to have a so-called "good time" at the expense of health and vitality, and the other way is to combine the pleasant with the useful!, i.e., not only have a pleasant time in the proper sense of the word, but also regain health and vigor, which have suffered more or less from the strain of the city life.

The many advantages which this resort offers to vacation guests are as follows:

It is located in one of the most healthy localities amidst the most beautiful country scenes and comprises sixty acres of ground, mostly woods and hills. The extensive grounds croquet, ball games, swimming and delightful excursions.

It cultivates a strictly homelike atmosphere and tolerates no objectionable features.

It is patronized by the better class of people. Children are at all times in good company and in no danger of associating with undesirable persons.

It has a good reputation for excellent home cooking. Guests also have an opportunity to go on a special diet, if they so desire.

Its sleeping cottages provide the most perfect ventilation.

It is not a place for style and luxury, but for simplicity, ease and comfort.

Its proximity to New York affords business men whose families are staying at the resort to go to town every day, or for a visit and recuperation, arrive on Friday or Saturday after business hours and remain over Sunday.

Its guests are assured of immediate attention by the resident physician in case of emergency.

Its rates are as moderate as at the average resort.

Prospective guests are cordially invited to come out and see our resort. A time table will be sent upon request. Trains leave from Erie R. R. Station in Jersey City. Take Hudson tunnel tube on any of Sixth Ave. Stations or from Hudson Terminal Station on Fulton St. Erie R. R. Ferries connect from W. 23d St. and Chambers St.

The Institution As A Winter Resort

Patients having a prejudice against taking the cure during the winter are probably not aware of the powerful effect of cold air upon the entire system.

There is no season of the year in which the air is purer and more invigorating than during the winter.

A patient undergoing a cure during the cold season will soon notice how quickly the appetite improves, how much better he digests and assimilates his food, how much more soundly he sleeps, how much stronger he feels and how much his personal appearance changes to his advantage in consequence.

No one need fear the cold as long as he is properly clothed and nourished.

That the treatments are adapted to the winter weather and greatly differ from those applied during the spring, summer and fall, is a matter of fact easily understood.

Rates

Preliminary Examination, $2 to...$5.00

For room, board, treatment and general Naturopathic attendance, $16 a week and $60 a month up

With massage or special manual treatments, $21 a week or $80 a month and up

For room and board for guests not taking treatments, $16.00 a week or $60.00 a month

For room, board and use of parks for transient guests........$2.50 a day

Single meals..50¢

All payments to be made weekly to monthly in advance

Carriage to or from Station...............................50¢

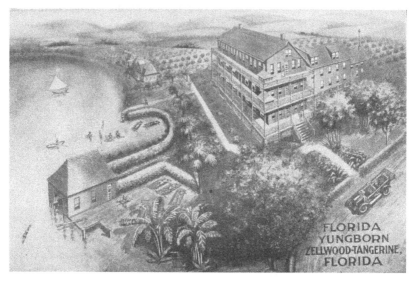

Dr. B. Lust's Recreation Resort "Florida Yungborg," Tangerine, Florida.

Symptoms are but the manifestation of the disease, not the disease itself, and to direct our efforts towards them, instead of their cause, is like chopping off the leaves of a weed to kill the plant.

The power that cures a disease lies in the patient himself. It is called the Vis Medicatrix Naturae, i.e., the inborn healing power which exists in every living body.

Without pure air there is no healthy blood, and without healthy blood there is no cure.

The Medical Trust Busy Again

by **R. E. Brandman**
The Naturopath and Herald of Health, XVIII(11), 723-725. (1913)

Action Is Absolutely Necessary. Another Owens Bill Came To Life.

In the House of Representatives September 27, 1913, the following bill, 8606 (by request) has been introduced by Mr. Reily of Connecticut:

"To create a United States Medical Licensing Board.

"Be it enacted by the Senate and House of Representatives of the United States of America in Congress assembled, that the President be, and he is hereby, authorized and directed to appoint two medical officers of the United States Army, with a rank of a captain and a major; two medical officers of the United States Navy, with a rank of lieutenant and lieutenant commander; and two medical officers of the United States Marine Hospital Corps, with rank of lieutenant and lieutenant commander to a board to be known as the United States Medical Licensing Board.

"Sec. 2. That the terms of the members of the board to be four years each, and the salary of each member thereof to be $4,000 per annum with mileage. Said board shall be in continuous session at Washington when not on duty in various States.

"Sec. 3. That all regular licensed medical practitioners of medicine, now holders of a medical diploma and a State license permitting them to practice in the respective States, shall upon the passage of this Act by presenting to said board their medical diploma, their State medical license, and any other diplomas they may have, and upon the payment of the sum of $2 be given a United States license which will permit them to practice their profession of medicine in any State or Territory of the United States and its possessions.

"Sec. 4. That the United States Licensing Board shall hold its meetings in various cities of the United States and shall examine all newly graduated medical doctors so that they may obtain a United States license, which license will permit them to practice medicine or surgery in any State or Territory of the United States and its possessions without any further examination: Provided, That the candidate for said license shall fulfill all the requirements of the American Medical Association and shall be an American citizen and present a high-school certificate or its equivalent and shall have a doctor of medicine diploma from a medical college in good standing, as declared by the American Medical Association, and upon payment of $10 and the filing of certificates of good moral character shall be admitted to examination and upon the passage of said examination shall be granted a United States license, which will permit the holder to practice medicine and surgery in any State or Territory of the United States and its possessions.

"Sec. 5. The license may be revoked in case abortions or other unprofessional and criminal acts are performed."

The bill was referred to the committee on Military Affairs and ordered to be printed. The bill is to **create a United States Medical Licensing Board** and ought to be vigorously opposed by every cult and by every one who believes in freedom and fair play. But like most bills which are of medical trust parentage, there is a sinister joker behind the published benevolent purpose of the proposed law. The doctors who are in charge of the political campaign of the Medical Trust know well enough that they cannot pass any such laws on their merits, so they always try to get their desires under cover of some worthy design. This is, however, characteristic of all trusts. It is well known that a larger percentage of the people believe in **Drugless Methods** more than they believe in the practice of regular medicine.

The regular system as taught and practiced by all compeers and as taught in the text-books in the medical schools, is untrue in philosophy, unfounded in nature, false in science, and absurd in practice; that it teaches a false doctrine of the essential nature of disease; a false doctrine of action of medicines; a false doctrine of the relations of disease to the living organism; a false doctrine of the relations of remedies to diseases;

a false theory of vitality; a false theory of this medicatrix naturae, or remedial power of nature, and a false doctrine of "nature's law of cure." All history attests the fact that wherever the Drug Medical System prevails, desolation marks its track, human health declines, vital stamina diminishes, diseases become more numerous, more complicated, and more fatal, and the human race deteriorates. Every drug taken into the living system induces a new disease, every drug has its own penalty, every dose is an outrage on the living system, and in disobedience to physiological law.

Look at Materia Medica of this false and fatal system once more. If you could see it but one instant with clear vision and unbiased mind, you would recoil from it with horror. You would renounce and execrate it forever.

What are its agents, its medicines, its remedies? Poisonous drugs and destructive processes. **Vaccines, toxines** [sic]**, serums,** scarifying, blistering, caustics, irritants, parasites, corrosives, minerals, vegetable excrescences and animal excretions, all of the causes of disease known to the three kingdoms of nature.

The effects of remedies are the phenomena of disease, and nothing else. We do indeed cure one disease by producing another.

How do medical men prove that these medicines are remedies for sick folks? In precisely the same way that toxicologists prove that they are poisons for well folks. When these remedies are given to well persons, they produce more or less nausea, vomiting, purging, pain, heat, swelling, griping, vertigo, spasms, stupor, coma, delirium and death. When they are given to sick persons, they produce the same manifestations of disease, modified more or less, by the condition of the patient and the circumstances of the prior disease. Was there ever any reasoning in the world like unto medical reasoning? If the medical man with good intentions administers one of these drug poisons, or a hundred of them, and the patient dies, he dies because the **medicine can't save him.** For one person injured by the use of patent medicines, one hundred have been destroyed by the doctors' prescriptions. For one person who has suffered loss by trusting to drugless methods who did nothing to relieve, there are hundreds who have been killed or maimed by reckless surgery. For one who has neglected to protect himself from contagion there are thousands who have been scared to death by the medical profession through needless alarm concerning contagion. For one who has died for the want of the right medicine at the right time one hundred have died as the result of the **wrong medicine at the wrong time.** I emphasize the fact that these are not my statements, but the statements of regular physicians who stand high in the medical profession. Pages, yes volumes, can be filled with such confessions from prominent members of the medical profession. Take them for what they are worth. If these are true it is time the people were finding it out. **The truth will hurt no honest man.**

Curing disease **without** drugs is a higher art than curing disease with drugs. He who shows that drugs are not necessary in a given class of cases is a benefactor to both humanity and the profession. Twenty-five million people want to see drugless methods have fair play and they would rise in their wrath if any Legislature should dare to attempt to suppress the practice. The only way to pass laws of real value is to pass them on their merits and not try to make them stalking horses for the usurpation of autocratic powers by some medical trust. When I speak thus of the medical trust, I do not attack the medical profession. I do not believe that **the rank and file** of the profession sanction such methods any more than the people of the United States sanction the way they have been sold out by their legislative representatives. The vast majority of real physicians are too ethical in their conduct and too broad-minded in their views to stoop to such contemptible political ways of crookedness. If the fate of Drugless Methods were left to the really scientific doctors, there would be little or nothing for the Drugless Doctor to fear. Does the Medical Trust fear for the people, or does it fear for itself? The Drug Medical System cannot bear examination. To explain it would be to destroy it, and to defend it even is to damage it.

What right has any body of men to prescribe another's choice as to what physician he or she shall employ, any more than to prescribe what church he or she shall attend? What right has the legislature to make laws to legalize the use of poison, under the pretence of it being a medicine? The right of choice is the strongest principle in the whole range of human action. The will of man as regards his own welfare is the most sacred right in all the realms of his physical existence, and for a law to be palmed off on the people just because a few poison venders formulate it, and lobby it through the legislative branches of the law-making powers, to satisfy the perverted malice upon designing men, is to perpetrate upon the people the grandest farce conceivable or imaginable. What do such enactments strike at? The very foundation of human liberty, the sacred rights of man to use the gifts or intelligence that God has endowed him with, and the skill which he himself has acquired. Such proceedings partake of the very nature of the "star chamber," whose decrees led to a revolution and the death of a great king of England on the scaffold. The very idea of there being such a thing – an Executionary Board – in any civilized state – a Medical Board, to control and regulate a set of poison venders, and to have their powers extended to ostracize everybody else who does not contribute to that gang! Where is the justice in legalizing a class of people to deal out poison to persons simply because they are diseased? While the masses are slow to act, slow to realize their privileges, yet, I venture to pre-dict that when the people learn that they can be cured without poisons introduced into their systems, the medical code of ethics, as it now is, will lose its influence, and the statute-makers will erase from its pages the disgraceful, unjust claw-law now on them. Man has four great enemies to fight: sickness, the Medical Trust, drugs, and the crude Osteopathic Trust. Instead of investigation, we find empiricism; instead of facts, we have theories; instead of correct conclusions, dogmatic rules; instead of ascertaining causes, we have useless talk. No science is so full of erroneous conclusions, mistakes, lies and dreams, as the so-called Science of Medicine and Osteopathy (may the Lord forgive them; they know not what they are doing).

As long as the medical and osteopathic profession continues to hunt bugs and attribute the diseases to them, advancement will be impeded, but when it is known that healthy blood excludes such a possibility, and that healthy blood results from normal circulation, they will cease their search for new bugs, or bug theories, and go to work to learn how to promote the normal circulation of the blood and other fluids of the body, in itself causing every disease known to mankind.

> Curing disease **without** drugs is a higher art than curing disease with drugs.
>
> Where is the justice in legalizing a class of people to deal out poison to persons simply because they are diseased?

A Message Of Health

by Benedict Lust

The Naturopath and Herald of Health, XVIII(11), 729-730. (1913)

Say, you who are ailing, have you reached the point where you are tired of doctoring? No, don't mistake. It is not the object of this article to recommend a new patent medicine nor any other medicine of any kind whatever. Perhaps you have tried several doctors one after the other and cheerfully swallowed the drugs the prescribed after solemnly declaring that their predecessor had been mistaken as to the nature of your ailment. After each new trial you felt better for a while and thought that at last you had found the proper remedy but afterwards the old trouble returned and you decided to try another doctor.

You don't need medicine of any kind. All drugs are harmful to the body in the long run. The fact that you have been taking medicine all this time and still are sick is proof enough of that. If on the other hand your complaint started recently, give Nature a chance before you begin letting the doctors dope you.

But to make use of the elements of Nature, you must live near to Nature while receiving treatment by the natural methods. In fact, natural living is part of the natural treatment. At the Yungborn, in the beautiful Ramapo Mountains, near Butler on the N. Y. Susquehanna and Western R. R. every facility is given to live the natural, open-air life and the institution is equipped with everything necessary for the natural treatment. There you may become again as a little child and run barefooted and care-free near laughing brooks, and through smiling valleys and over rugged mountains. By means of external water treatment, living in the open air, sun, light and air baths, under the direction of competent assistants, and proper and natural diet, wonderful cures are being effected every day. Don't you know that hundreds of people who, perhaps like yourself, had taken drugs and changed doctors until they were discouraged are being radically cured now-a-days by the elements of pure nature properly applied?

Stop taking medicine; cut it all out. If you haven't taken it yet, don't begin. Come out to the Yungborn and be cured by Nature herself, and enjoy yourself at the same time. Be cured in the way God meant you to be cured, in the way His creatures of the forest and the field cure themselves.

Stop and think for a minute. Why is it that animals enjoy such robust bodily health and strength, and that among them, the wild animals, those who live in the freedom of forest and jungle, are more hardy than those domesticated animals which live within the confines of so-called civilization and are subject to some of its effeminating influences? Why is it that the wounded animal immediately rushes to the woods and seeks the water? How do animals live? In the first place, they live continually out of doors, they breathe always the pure, fresh air, at night as well as in the day time, they eat the food that Nature provides for them and their instinct leads them to choose, they bathe in the streams and rivers, the recline and rest on the ground in the bright sunlight or in the cool shade of the trees and in consequence their bodies are filled with the energy and vitality that they absorb continually from the earth, the sun the air and the water. If you would become strong and hardy and robust as they are, you must adopt something of their mode of life.

Return to Nature. Sweet Nature hold out her hands to you filled with her gifts of sparkling health and strength if you will but approach her in confidence and partake of them. She calls to you from the woods and fields, the meadows and brooks, the wild flowers that bloom on the mountain side and the stately trees that wave in the forest. Her voice is in the song of the birds that rings with joy and gladness in the morning hours in the tinkling of the cool stream that winds its way over the pebbly bottom through the shady woods, in the loving of the cows at evening in the distant pasture and the sighing of the breeze through the leafy boughs.

I tell you the forces that fill these things with life, can impart life and energy and health to your own body. Be done with drugs and medicines. Come to Nature and let her cure you in her own way.

If you have never heard of the wonderful success of the natural method of treatment by the proper use of the elements of Nature, water, sun, earth and air, write to us for further information. Or better still run out to the Yungborn some day and look the place over. There are many trains daily and it only takes a little over an hour from Jersey City to Butler. The Yungborn is only about a mile from the village, right up in the mountains. Everybody in Butler can tell you just where it is. You can get a carriage at the station if you wish. Come out and enjoy the scenery and the change and learn how you can get well in a delightful and pleasant way, amid charming surroundings and without drugs or medicines.

Return to Nature. Sweet Nature hold out her hands to you filled with her gifts of sparkling health and strength if you will but approach her in confidence and partake of them. She calls to you from the woods and fields, the meadows and brooks, the wild flowers that bloom on the mountain side and the stately trees that wave in the forest. Her voice is in the song of the birds that rings with joy and gladness in the norming hours in the tinkling of the cool stream that winds its way over the pebbly bottom through the shady woods, in the loving of the cows at evening in the distant pasture and the sighing of the breeze through the leafy boughs.

1914

NATUROPATHIC LEGISLATION SERIES:
PART ONE: BRIEF I, II, AND III

NY STATE SOCIETY OF NATUROPATHS

Subscription advertisement, *The Naturopath and Herald of Health*, April 1914, XIX(4).

Naturopathic Legislation Series:
Part One: Brief I, II, and III

NY State Society of Naturopaths
The Naturopath and Herald of Health, XIX(3), 143-150. (1914)

BRIEF I

Reasons For The Passing Of A Naturopathic Law

As citizens, voters and taxpayers of this state, we have an inalienable right to participate in the making and conducting of this Government and Legislature. In this State, since the year 1896, some five hundred drugless practitioners have been engaged in practice, using the so called natural methods of healing, such as hydrotherapy, light and air cure, diet, physical culture, Swedish movements and other systems of manipulation of the body. The institutions conducted by these natural healers were generally patronized by men and women, whose health and strength had given way to disease, or such as were bodily and mentally exhausted from over-work or other causes, and their restoration was uniformly brought about by rational methods of cure and by teaching them how to live and avoid the causes of disease. The underlying principle of these drugless methods of healing is prophylaxis or prevention of disease by right living and the acquiring of normal habits, conforming to the laws of nature which underlie all things.

The laws have been amended over and over again by the actions of the different medical societies, and gradually these amendments have brought into existence a system of laws on our statue-books under which practically and virtually everything done for the preservation or restoration of health constitutes medical practice, or a misdemeanor.

We have the proofs to show that a large number of hydropathic or nature-cure institutions have been ruined and broken up, and people who were engaged in the practicing of these drugless methods of curing and preventing diseases were driven out of the State. In some instances, men and women thus engaged were arrested, convicted and condemned to long prison sentences and to the payment of heavy fines, suffering almost inconceivable hardship and loss under the persecution of this medical trust combination. It is also a fact that the fines collected by these proceedings are to a great extent used by these medical societies as a means for continuing actively the persecution of the drugless practitioners. Thus men and women who were guilty of no other offense than the giving of a bath or a massage, the instruction in dietetics or systems of exercise, were heavily and unmercifully fined or sent to jail. In some instances, the officers of the New York Country Medical Society called on the proprietors of these nature-cure institutions or graft, and when such tribute was refused, they would send spies and sleuths, who by any means, fair or foul and under any pretense would work up a case against them; as for instance, the giving of a bath was held up in court as a violation of the medical law, and the proprietor of the bathing establishment and the attending nurse were fined $200.00. In many instances it has been proven that these emissaries of this medical trust were of a doubtful character, and that they without scruple or hesitation committed perjury, and convictions were obtained on the strength of such false or perjured statements.

This condition has become unbearable. There is no reason why the people of the State of New York should not have at their service practitioners of drugless methods of healing and nature-cure institutions, when they want them-and they have shown that they do want them. As the law stands today, the citizen who believes in drugless methods, cannot lawfully secure such relief, and is forced to take drugs, even though he has no faith whatsoever in these merits. This is a violation of the constitutional rights of these citizens of this state, quite apart from the fact that drugless practitioners or Naturopaths by practical test and demonstration have proven their ability to cure where other methods absolutely failed.

We are in position to prove by the records of actual cases, that positive cure, permanent restoration to health and strength, was brought about where medical doctors had given up the patients as lost.

Nature-Cure or Naturopathy is now recognized in every civilized country of the world, and there is no good reason why it should not enjoy the recognition and protection of the State of New York, as well as any other system of healing by drugs or old school methods. This new school, established for the relief and prevention of disease has come to stay. It is a fact that every advance which during the past three centuries has been made in the prevention and cure of disease, were the work of laymen. Medical trust-doctors uniformly opposed such advances as long as they could, and then when they found that the public really wanted them, they incorporated it in their own systems and appropriated them as their own.

From an economic, social and moral standpoint alike, drugless methods for the prevention and cure of disease are justifiable in this and every other state. Wherever these methods are practiced, they invariably raise the standard of manhood and womanhood, teach the people how to keep healthy and strong without recourse to drugs, encourage them to live a simple life, comforting to the laws of health and hygiene, and how to acquire wholesome, health-giving habits.

This, in brief, is the argument upon which we respectfully plead that you give us your kind cooperation and assistance towards the passing of bill 281.

Respectfully,
NEW YORK STATE SOCIETY OF NATUROPATHS

BRIEF II

PRACTICAL IDEALS EMBODIED IN NATUROPATHY

Twentieth century Therapeutics should make it their principal object and purpose to re-establish the union of man's body, brain, heart and all bodily functions- with nature. This purpose can only be accomplished by a right understanding of the laws which operate throughout all living things in nature, and to this end the following methods of Naturopathy are found useful and indispensable,- each in its own place, time and preferment:

DIETETICS

HYDROTHERAPY

PHYSICAL CULTURE

DYNAMIC BREATHING

MASSAGE

SWEDISH MOVEMENTS

STRUCTURAL ADJUSTMENT

SUN

LIGHT

AIR BATHS

KNEIPP CURE

JUST CURE

FASTING

And such other simple natural agencies as REST, WORK, REC-REATION, SUGGESTION, VIBRATION, etc. NATURE CURE is a system of man-building harmonizing with constructive principles of Nature, conforming to the physical, mental, moral and spiritual planes of being. The constructive principles of nature are those which build up, improve and repair, always working toward and having as their ideal the most uniformly perfect type - the type which of all has survived in the evolutionary process, as opposed to the destructive forces of nature to which the weaker types succumbed.

NATUROPATHY makes it our business to discover and bring out whatever latent strength and purpose any one individual may possess, to encourage, strength, harden and vitalize it against the disintegrating, destroying forces, until a balance in favor of the constructive principle is struck.

HEALTH is in reality nothing more or less than harmonious adjustment and vibration of the component elements of being, including physical, mental, moral and spiritual planes. In other words, constructive principle applied to individual life.

DISEASE is abnormal or inharmonious vibration of the same component elements of being, as related to the same physical, mental, moral and spiritual planes.

THE PRIMARY CAUSE OF DISEASE, barring accident or surgical injury to the human organism, or a hostile, destructive environment, is VIOLATION OF NATURE'S LAWS. The effect following any and all violations of the immutable laws of nature is, primary and principally, lowered vitality, an abnormal composition of blood and lymph, accumulation of waste matter in the body—a poisoning of the well-springs of the organism.

These conditions are identical with what is known as disease. The Naturopathic methods of cure are made to conform closely to the constructive principles of natural law, and we recognize as such:

FIRST—The establishment of normal, moral surroundings and natural habits of life to conform with natural laws.

SECOND—An economizing of the vital forces and the increasing and rejuvenating of these by any means known to science.

THIRD—A reconstruction of the blood to conform to a sound, normal, natural basis; in other words, a supplying of the blood with its natural constituents in correct proportion, to produce that bodily harmony which is known as health.

FOURTH—To promote and facilitate the elimination of the waste matters and poisons that are injurious and destructive to the human organism.

FIFTH—An arousing in the individual of the highest possible degree of consciousness and sense of personal accountability, making him realize that supreme importance of intelligent sustained personal effort, or self-help.

WE RECOGNIZE MEDICINES as being in conformity with the constructive principles of nature in so far as they are harmless and non-destructive to the human organism and act as tissue foods or promote the neutralization and elimination of morbid matters and poisons. POISONOUS DRUGS OR PERNICIOUS OPERATIONS conform to the destructive principles of nature because they halt or suppress the natural run of the disease and precipitate natural reaction (The crisis). They interfere with the harmonious cleansing and healing efforts of nature and thus become injurious and destructive to human life in more sense than one—(both as poisons and meddlers with natural course). Moreover, such treatment is harmful by the fact that it engenders the belief that it can be substituted for the recognition of and obedience to nature's immutable laws. It fosters the false and fatal impression in the patient's mind that he may by the grace of powder and pills evade personal responsibility—that intelligent self-help and effort are unnecessary and may be substituted by drugs.

NATUROPATHY has come to take the place of such drugs and schools because it teaches that the primary and underlying cause of all disease, barring such agents as we indicated above, is violation of the laws of nature. By an awakening in the patient of the realization of this great truth an interest is created in him to consider and know intelligently every law and agent in nature which operates for health or disease, construction or destruction, of his bodily and mental functions. Thuswise it arouses and strengthens the sense of personal responsibility in the individual, as related to his own immediate state of health, to the hereditary conditions of his life which confront him and to his duty to posterity through his offspring.

NATUROPATHY, then, makes claim for recognition because:

IT ENCOURAGES PERSONAL EFFORT AND SELFHELP. IT SEEKS TO ADAPT ENVIRONMENT AND HABITS OF LIFE TO CONFORM TO NATURAL LAW.

IT ASSISTS NATURE'S CLEANSING AND HEALING EFFORTS.

ITS MEANS AND METHODS OF TREATMENT ARE HARMLESS, SIMPLE AND WITHIN EVERYBODY'S REACH. IT POINTS THE WAY TO A NATURAL METHOD OF LIVING AS REGARDS EATING, DRINKING, BREATHING, BATHING, DRESSING, WORKING, RESTING, THINKING, MORALITY.

Our object and purpose now and always will be to bring humanity back to a rational, normal, natural basis of living, to regulate, as far as it is in our power, the sexual, social and moral life of the patient who comes to us for help, through such agents as have been indicated herein.

WE HOLD vaccination, vivisection, poisonous drugs, gluttony, intoxication and the likes to be abhorrent to nature and destructive to the well-being, health and happiness of mankind.

WE BELIEVE that to the development of healthy, happy life and the best type of man is necessary a recognition of the principles we have embodied in NATUROPATHY, making for an incessant unfoldment of inner perception, purpose and knowledge together with the systemic development of visible outer power, so that through such conscious development and intelligent sustained effort the individual may at length be fully and harmoniously expressed and the highest possible type of mortal being always arrived at.

WE HAVE LEARNED that simplicity in everything offers the clear-est clue to salvation, physical, mental and material. That the survival of the fittest struggle, governing civilization is from physical to men-tal, from mental (just now) to financial, but from financial back to the spiritual. That to find the well-spring of bountiful health or exuberant, exhilarating joy, man must first find himself and his powers by diligent effort and sustained application.

That one of the primal essentials toward a healthy, happy life is and always will be the love of somebody or some noble ideal more than one's own ease and well-being and, thus loving and aspiring, forgetting the things which lie behind, whose joys or sorrows, hopes or fears are gone forever, and reaching out for the endless future with its boundless possibilities for greater and greater unfoldment, knowledge and power.

Such are the motives and ideals with which we come before the world and ask for recognition; and that our school be justly judged as opposed to that of Allopathy, the obsolete school of medical science (?) which, as is well known, reasons not from the underlying cause, not from fundamental principle, but from external symptoms, personal experience and surface effects. It is our mission to bring home to mankind the fact that this school of healing (?), full of errors, bungling, doubts, confusion and hit-and-miss methods is a failure.

OR HAVE A LOOK AROUND YOU AND SEE IF IT IS NOT?

Respectfully yours,
NEW YORK STATE SOCIETY OF NATUROPATHS

BRIEF III

AN APPEAL FROM THE CITIZENSHIP OF NEW YORK TO THE GOVERNOR, SENATE AND ASSEMBLY

A failure on the part of the licensed medical profession to successfully administer to the requirements and necessities of the citizen of N.Y. in his sickness and infirmities is equivalent to the sentence of death, from the positive and absolute fact that the Medical Board Law debars said citizen from every other therapeutic means of relief practiced in the State, after which said citizen has no legal alternative for life but to leave the State and go beyond the dominion of said law where other rational and efficient therapeutic means are tolerated by the law of the land.

Is the State giving the individual rights of the citizen proper consideration when said citizen is driven to the extremely embarrassing but positive emergency of requiring another citizen to commit an act which is violation of the Criminal Laws of the State, in order to secure such attention and assistance as is absolutely essential to the protection of the health and life of the citizen.

Our State and County Officials are doing this every day in our State. Will the Legislature relieve her citizens of this embarrassing situation?

It is fact that the people are obtaining relief through naturopathic methods. How can it be otherwise when such results are gladly acknowledged by the people we live among, our very neighbors, men and women we meet face to face every day, some of which are well-known in the very sections where they utterly failed to obtain a cure or relief from the medical profession?

1915

EFFICIENCY IN DRUGLESS HEALING

EDWARD EARLE PURINTON

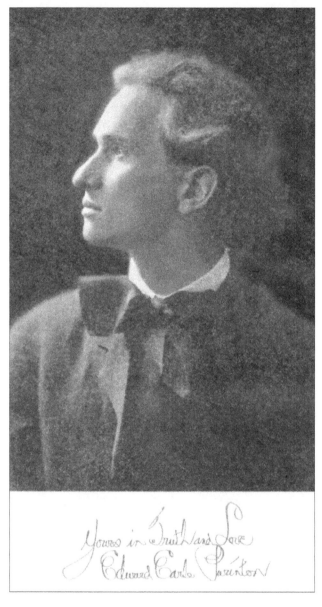

Edward Earle Purinton.

Efficiency In Drugless Healing

by Edward Earle Purinton

The Naturopath and Herald of Health, XX(1), 1-7. (1915)

A YEAR OF TRIUMPH

A Happy New Year—the happiest of all that have come and gone, with gains and blessings, human and divine, showered more upon you every day. This is my earnest wish for every friend and comrade who reads this magazine.

But wishing is not enough—I don't stop here. The people who only wish for things are lazy beyond redeem. Rule for success: Want something so hard you'll break your neck going after it. Then, even if you don't get it, you will be satisfied; for, having broken your neck, you won't need it any more. Be a crusader of some kind—any kind—if you really want to *live*. Most people, being made of mush, deserve to sizzle.

I am going to tell you, hygienic neighbor, how to ensure a happy New Year for yourself by *earning* it. And there is no other way to get it. Believe me, any man or woman who carries out a fraction of the plan suggested in the forthcoming articles, will have to be an angel in wisdom, strength, goodness. And are not angels happy?

Few practitioners of drugless methods are ever downright happy. Their whole career is one long fight. Their toil, devotion, courage, faith, sacrifice deserve the richest rewards that life can bestow. Yet some are languishing in prison, others have been martyred, others are facing daily persecution, all for the sake of principle.

We can have a great new year of triumph. But we've got to change some of our methods. They have been methods of failure. And it will take all the resolution we can muster, plus a deal of humility and grace, to look the situation in the eye.

When you probe for a bullet, you can't stop to ask the patient if he likes the feel of your knife. We have all been grievously wounded by the missiles of the Medical Trust. In these articles I am probing for bullets—searching out the sore spots and the weak spots—trying to save our life by opening up the wounds. We all need a mental surgeon, to show us our vulnerable spot. And even though it is a thankless job, I am here to carry it through.

When a great army finds itself on the wrong track, what does it do? Takes to cover. Then, having reconnoitered, provisioned itself and shaped its course anew, it plows ahead with the dauntless force of supreme faith. In a thousand-and-one ways, more or less, we have been on the wrong track. The airship has become the international scout in war; so I am hoping that these articles may form a kind of mental airship, from which we may gain a clearer view of the opposing camp, and of our own strategic position.

Our first great need is to unite all the forces of drugless therapeutics under a single banner, with a single purpose, on a single method. How can this be done?

Let us examine the situation. We have, I should judge, at least 100 different schools and schemes of health in America, all condemning the use of drugs. These various methods run the gamut of psychology and physiology, from the Christian Science to Massage. Each has some truth, none has all truth. Each is a logical branch of department of a great central system, uniting and co-ordinating them all. Doctor B. Lust calls this central system Naturopathy—you may call it anything you please, if you only recognize the basic truth of it.

Now let me give you a scientific reason why the various bills before legislatures, arguing for the license of drugless healers, have not been passed. Of course the apparent reason is the opposition of the medical fraternity; but the *real* reason is something very different. Let us take for example the Christian Science bill and the Mechano-Therapy bill recently proposed at Albany. Neither of these bills, in my opinion, ever should be passed by any State legislature. If they were passed, without revision and a central supervision, they would be a menace to health and liberty—as constant a menace as the drug-laden laws of the past have become!

In the light of logic and jurisprudence, there is no more reason to license a healer who gives manipulations or suggestions than to license a doctor who gives drugs. The only test for both is efficiency: What does each *know,* what can each *do?* Some day—some day far off—when we are beginning to be civilized, we will pass a law like this: Every candidate for a doctor's degree and license shall be required to diagnose, treat and cure a certain number of cases of disease, both chronic and acute, and sufficiently diverse to cover the points in the average daily practice; he shall gain a certain percentage of successful cures, and shall submit references to corroborate the cures, before a license may be granted him to practice indiscriminately.

We will have, in short, a doctor's apprentice school, as we now have a barber's apprentice school. Why should a doctor be allowed to kill under State license—when a barber is not allowed to cut your chin? The doctor's apprentice school will grant diplomas irrespective of drug or anti-drug theories of its students. The question will be simply: "Can you cure this disease—quickly, safely, permanently? If so, you may hang out your shingle. If not, the shingle will be applied to that section of your anatomy where bad boys have learned to look for it." When I get to be President of the United States, I shall introduce a law creating an official spanking-machine for unsuccessful doctors. When they have buried five patients, they shall be gorgeously dressed in high-hat and broad-cloth, then conducted by automobile and a brass band to the town spanking-machine, and be gently labored with, in full view of the assembled populace. This measure, while somewhat lacking in dignity, would be redolent of honesty.

Pardon the digression; when I start to think of the doctor-business, my risibles run off with me.

Let us return to the Mechano-Therapy and Christian Science bills before the legislature. By no means would I charge the lawmakers of our State with trying to be public benefactors;—manifestly they are not guilty. But I do thank them for preventing the passage of any measure to hurt our cause in the end—no matter if their veto is a signature of shame. For without question, the legalizing of any single branch of the Nature Cure would react badly on the whole movement.

Please remember that Doctor Lust is not responsible for my opinions—in fact he often disagrees with them. But we both are seeking truth, just as you are. And all sides must be heard.

A confusion of thought is the beginning of all our troubles. Let us see how. If you have a chronic ailment, such as liver trouble or asthma, you go to a Christian Scientist, and are given a certain diagnosis and treatment. Next day you consult a Mechano-Therapist, and for the same disease you get a wholly different diagnosis and treatment. Which is right? Both cannot be right. Which *is* right?

We accuse the doctors of "guess-work." We are guilty of it ourselves. They guess with drugs, we guess without drugs. That is the only difference between us.

Each of the hundred branches of drugless healing in America wants to be legalized—and no one deserves to be. We have all got the cart before the horse, we have to put license ahead of merit. Authority is the echo of capacity; and if God Almighty wanted us to practice without restraint, He would enact a Pentecost or a Sinai, and force our law through, in spite of ten thousand bribed and chained legislators.

The question for us to answer is this: Does Christian Science, or New Thought, or Massage, or Diet, or Hydropathy, *cure?* I have known cases where every single form of natural treatment failed to cure, despite the allegations and promises of all the different healers. And I have known of the most absurd claims by fanatical zealots; that even a child, not half-witted, would smile at.

An Osteopath offered to cure by a few turns of the hand a case of extreme nervous exhaustion due to long years of anxiety, over-work and underfeeding. A chiropractor wanted to take a man from the operating-table when gangrene from appendicitis had set in; the Chiropractor was sure he could waft the gangrene away, by a set of magical passes. An eloquent masseur guaranteed to grow hair on a bald head, when the roots had all come out. And a bejewelled high-priestess of metaphysical rot said she could think a lady's hump-backed nose into becoming a work of art. With such fakers in our midst, unmolested and unrebuked, how can we hope for a State license to do anything worth while? Some doctors are charlatans—and we are all chumps. The variation isn't much to crow over.

Doubtless you have seen what befell among the Osteopaths. Ten years ago they were with us heart and soul in our fight against medical tyranny. Now they have largely withdrawn the hand of fellowship, choosing instead the hand of finance. The Osteopaths are today almost as much a close corporation as the allopaths—a bit of legal standing has made them highly bumptious and domineering. And the Mechano-therapist or Mental Scientist or Dietist or Physcultopathist would behave just as foolishly under a similar premature State license. It is just as ridiculous to legalize any of them as it would be to elect a college professor from a class of boys who had just learned the alphabet. Not one of them knows enough to be given a doctor's license.

Here somebody stands up in meeting and shouts angrily, wanting to know since when have I become a traitor to the cause? Be calm, neighbor, and remember that truth is never reached by a man in a temper. I have never been so real a friend of Nature Cure and Mind Cure as I am at this moment; but instead of shooting a volley of words all over creation and hitting nothing—as the majority of drugless healers do—I have learned to train a battery of *deeds* on the walls of my ambition, which walls were crumbling and I am entering the breastworks. The trouble with the anti-drug forces is, they use their mouths too much and their brains too little. Valuable suggestion to reformers: A holler is a poor substitute for a headpiece.

Our whole fight has been conducted on wrong lines. This I expect to prove to any fair-minded man, before I get through with this series of articles. Meanwhile be patient—we must start from the beginning. If I said now what I shall finally say, you might fall in such a rage you would get the blind staggers, which would interfere with your sight, and all my effort would be wasted. That would not be efficiency, now would it?

The great obstacle to the advancement of the Nature Cure in America is well shown by a recent conversation with a health reformer in a prominent position among the foes of medicine. The substance of his remarks went thusly: "I approve the work you are doing, to wake us all up, and am in hearty sympathy with the aims of Naturopathy. But I cannot join a movement that allows such fellows as Doctor Jones and Healer Smith to have a place in it. Doctor Jones is merely a bone-setter, and Healer Smith a crazy believer in the occult. My system of original manipulations is the only scientific mode of treatment, therefore you must bar Doctor Jones and Healer Smith from the practice of Naturopathy, or ask no support from me."

Having heard the opinion of this gentleman, whom we will call Professor Brown, I went to Doctor Jones for advice in the matter. Doctor Jones agreed with Professor Brown regarding the merits of Naturopathy, but said Professor Brown ran a fake school and should not be encouraged in his vileness. Being somewhat bewildered, I bethought me to get from Healer Smith a really unprejudiced view of the controversy. Healer Smith said Naturopathy was all right, but why for goodness' sake did we associate with such a liar as Professor Brown and such a quack as Doctor Jones?

I ask you, speaking from the heart out, what can we do with such a gang of goops? This is our real problem.

There are just two fundamental principles on which we can unite with all the practitioners, patrons and friends of rational healing methods. Neither of these principles regards the merits of any one system as compared with any other; and only by taking and enforcing such a neutral position can we ever join hands. The two basic principles are these:

1. Every grown, sane citizen has a right to choose his own doctor.
2. Drugs are always injurious, often dangerous, and never to be used when a natural means will effect a cure.

The Mechano-Therapist and the Christian Scientist heartily agree on these two propositions. Then why do they not take their stand on this common ground, to wage a holy war against the drug and knife? Suppose the right wing of the German army had said, "We will use only bullets"; and the left wing had said, "We will use only swords"; and the main host had said, "We will use only prayers";—how long would the German army have lasted? Union, concentration, perfect knowledge of a central system, training in a central school, obedience to a central authority, made the German army equal to France, England and Russia put together. For the Christian Scientist or the Mechano-Therapist to strike out alone is as fatal as it would be for a single regiment to challenge a whole army of enemies; and with absurd ease have the allies of the doctors, druggists and undertakers killed off these single movements, one after another.

By a conservative estimate, hundreds of thousands of dollars would have been saved through a scientific union of all drugless practitioners. For example, I know a great hygienic pioneer who has lost $10,000 because of persecution by the Medical Trust. After years of suffering—mental, financial and social—he has worked out a system of blocking the medical sleuths and spies, avoiding arrest and escaping unjust fines. The original system of parrying the sneaks has been worth at least $1,000 a year to the man who works it. Suppose now that he were a member of a national association reaching every drugless doctor in America; and that he could mail the particulars of his secret method to each member of the association;—what a godsend this would be, how much energy, money and anxiety it would save to all the health reformers!

Today, every man who tries to help his fellows on and up to freedom goes through martyrdom, because he must make his own mistakes with no means of learning from the mistakes of his predecessors. Tomorrow, a central clearing-house will have been established, where daily reports of progress from all over the United States will be received, filed, culled, copied and distributed; and where every healer in search of help or advice may be sure of commanding the support that he needs.

This great union to come will be so broad, shrewd and sympathetic that the psychic and the masseur—wonder of wonders—will lock arms and call each other good fellows; and that the Osteopath, when the Christian Scientist is wrongly treated, will rise up in a huge wrath, to smite the invader of his hygienic household.

The union will forbid all criticism and condemnation of the physicians, whether drugfull or drugless; and will impose a fine on the member who speaks or writes in opposition to the rule.

It will occupy itself entirely with constructive work, wasting no time nor strength in the folly of battle. Having secured thousands of attested cases of cure by drugless means, it will base its appeal on facts alone—a kind of argument that is unanswerable, but that has never yet been used in our struggle for sanction by the law.

It will compile a directory of all healers, teachers, publishers, and manufacturers throughout America; and will adopt a system of credentials, based on a high standard of qualifications, whereby the many brands of quack and ignoramus in our fold may be separated from the few leaders that are capable and worthy.

It will spend its force not on militarism against the old-style doctors, but on the arrest, prosecution and eviction of the hundreds of so-called drugless healers who are a disgrace to our calling.

It will standardize the schools and health homes and sanitaria, as the Carnegie Foundation has already standardized hundreds of academic institutions; so that when a health system bears the seal of approval of association, every possible client or student or customer may know he is safe in spending time and money here.

It will maintain a corps of attorneys, editors, financial advisers and efficiency engineers, for the benefit of all its members; and will supply any service needed at cost price, from writing a good form letter and printing an effective booklet, to raising money for a hospital or chartering a health university.

My dream of the great achievement of such splendid union goes much further. But you have enough to think about. May I suggest that you write Doctor Lust the results of your thought? A mental union must precede an organic union, and a free discussion of these articles will make for increased efficiency on all sides. Am I wrong? If so, how? Am I right? Then what are you going to *do* about it? My part in helping to make this new year one of triumph is to rouse thought and feeling

Advertisement, December 1915, *The Naturopath and Herald of Health*, XX (12).

on the points that seem most vital. Your part is to *act,* promptly and decisively, on the suggestion that most appeals to you.

The first logical move is to join the two or three national associations of hygienists and drugless physicians that contain the possibilities of endless good. Will you not ask Doctor Lust for their names and addresses, write for their literature, and start to get in line for the mutual benefits of scientific organization?

Our first great need is to unite all the forces of drugless therapeutics under a single banner, with a single purpose, on a single method. How can this be done?

By a conservative estimate, hundreds of thousands of dollars would have been saved through a scientific union of all drugless practitioners.

1916

The History Of The Healing Art In The Progress Of Drugless Therapy

Wallace Fritz, M.D., D.D.S., N.D., D.O., D.C.

An Open Letter By Dr. B. Lust To The Drugless Profession Of The United States Of America

Benedict Lust

Neuropathy Department

Address all communications for this department to its editor

W. WALLACE FRITZ, M.D., D.D.S., N.D., 1600 Summer St., Philadelphia, Pa.

Professor of Neuropathy and Dean in the American College of Neuropathy, and President of the National Association of Drugless Physicians

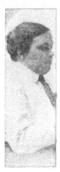

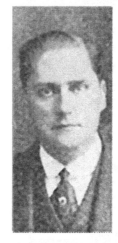

ASSOCIATE EDITOR:

SARAH E. GROVES, N.D.

Professor of Physiology in the Am. College of Neuropathy and Secretary of the National Association of Drugless Physicians

1113 Spruce St., Phila., Pa.

ASSOCIATE EDITOR:

THOMAS M. JACKSON, D.D., N.D.

Professor of Anatomy in the American College of Neuropathy

1533 Diamond St., Phila., Pa.

THE HISTORY OF THE HEALING ART IN THE PROGRESS OF DRUGLESS THERAPY

By Wallace Fritz, M. D., D. D. S., N. D., D. O., D. C.

Presidents address at the convention of the National Association of Drugless Practitioners, held at Atlantic City, N. J., June 1915.

Address by Wallace Fritz at the convention of the National Association of Drugeless Practitioners, held at Atlantic City, N.J., June 1915.

The History Of The Healing Art In The Progress Of Drugless Therapy

by Wallace Fritz, M.D., D.D.S., N.D., D.O., D.C.

Herald of Health and the Naturopath, XXI(1), 26-29. (1916)

Presidents Address At The Convention Of The National Association Of Drugless Practitioners, Held At Atlantic City, N. J., June 1915

In the 19th century Anesthesia (the Nitrous oxide or laughing gas) and different forms of serum treatment were introduced. (Dr. Jenner was the first one to advocate the use of Vaccine Virus for smallpox in 1798). "The lancet was the indispensable adjunct of the physician and that calomel, ipecac, squills, tartar-emetic, castor oil and senna were given for almost any ill." Also, that about one hundred years ago, (1803) patients who were convalescing from a fever were ordered a diet consisting of soup made from frogs, reptiles, snails and other loathsome creatures.

During the latter part of the 19th Century different systems of Drugless Therapy were introduced as Christian Science, Osteopathy, Chiropractory, Spondylo-Therapy, etc. In the early part of the 20th Century, Neuropathy was advanced by the writer as the most scientific method of the healing art up to the present.

The Eclectic School of Medicine was founded by Agathinus, of Sparta, about 90 A.D. This sect, which was closely allied to the "Phneumatists" avoided theories and metaphysical speculations, and selected from all the proceeding systems of medicine the opinions that seemed to them to be most reasonable and beneficial. Dr. Alexander Wilder says that of the ancient times, "The Eclectic School abounded with physicians of marked ability, many of them enjoyed a wide reputation over the Roman world, nor did it die out until political and other changes had produced a general revolution over the Empire."

Electrism was revived, when in 1845, "The Eclectic Medical Institute of Cincinnati" was incorporated, and in the announcement of its foundation the following statement was published.

Our College will be strictly what its name indicates—Eclectic— excluding all such medicines and such remedies as 'under the ordinary circumstances of their judicious use, are liable to produce evil consequences, or endanger the future health of the patient', while we draw from any and every source all such medicines and modes of treating disease as are found to be valuable, and at the same time, not necessarily attended with bad consequences.

At a meeting of the National Eclectic Medical Association held in Rochester, N. Y., in 1852, the following "platform of principles" was laid down:

1. "The first proposition was to maintain the utmost freedom of thought and investigation, in opposition to the restrictive system heretofore in vogue."

2. "To encourage the cultivation of Medical Science in a liberal spirit, especially in the development of resources of the vegetable Materia Medica, and the safest, speediest and most efficient methods of treating diseases."

3. "To adopt in investigations the Baconian or inductive philosophy instead of the synthetic methods."

4. "That a departure from the healthy condition interrupts the bodily functions, and only the recuperative efforts of Nature can effect their restoration. The object, therefore, of medication accordingly is to afford to Nature the same means of doing this work more advantageously, and under circumstances in which she would otherwise fall."

5. "To receive and teach Eclecticism—not as an indiscriminate selection of means supposed to be remedial, but a selection based upon the recognized nature of the disease to be treated, and the character of the agent or agents employed to remove that disease, thus presupposing a knowledge on the part of the physician, at one of the pathology of the disease and the adaptedness of the remedy, and to encourage and urge the highest scientific attainments."

6. "The excluding of all permanently depressing and disorganizing agencies—such as depletion by the lancet, and medication of a dangerous tendency; also preferring of vegetable remedies, but no exclusive system of Herbalism—and of a mineral agent, except from the conviction of its injurious effect."

7. "To dismiss from the catalogue of remedial agents all those which under circumstances of their administration are liable to injure the stamina of the human constitution; more particularly the mineral poisons, such as mercury, arsenic, and antimony, and all of their various preparations, and to substitute in their place articles derived from the vegetable kingdom, which are not only as powerful in their operation, but are more safe and salutary in their immediate effects upon the human system."

Rosewell Park says:

"The true eclectic recognizes no rule than his particular taste, reason, or fancy, and two or more eclectics have little or nothing in common. If that were true two thousand years ago, it is not much less to-day. The eclectic carefully avoids the discussion of principles, and has neither taste or capacity for abstract reasoning, although he may be a good practitioner; not that he has no ideas, but that his ideas form no working system. With his medical tact—i.e., cultivated instinct—replaces principles."

"The eclectic of our day, however, is only an empiric in disguise, that is, a man whose theoretical ideas do not go beyond phenomena." True eclecticism in medicine, however, it is individualism existed into fixed principles, or, as Renonard says, it is individuals, erected into a dogma, which escapes refutation because it is deficient in principles.

The Thomson treatment [was] founded by Samuel Thomson who was born in New Hampshire, in 1769. He discarded the lancet, leech, cupping-glass and Spanish fly, and the various mineral drugs, generally in use, substituting instead, medicines consisting of roots and herbs, which the members of this sect themselves prepared, the roots being dried and powdered, while the herbs were made into infusions, tinctures, and extracts which were concentrated and made into pills.

"Gorton" writes that Thomson divided diseases and their remedies into two classes—hot and cold—his theory being that "heat is life and cold is death." So that in cold stages of fever he prescribed hot drinks; and in the hot stages of fever and inflammations he gave cooling drinks. In cases of pneumonia or pleurisy, ipecac, or lobelia in mild doses was added as expectorant.

Regarding the Thomsonian treat—the stomach was considered the organ upon whose proper action depends almost entirely the maintenance of heat and health; therefore, the main indication in the treatment of disease is the clearing out of the stomach and its restoration to proper action; this was accomplished by violent euretics [sic]. Also; "The influence of torpidity of the excretory functions, especially of the perspiration, in causing disease, was recognized."

In Thomson's own words:

"That all diseases are the effect of one general cause and may be removed by one general remedy, is the foundation upon which I have erected my fabric."

He has peculiar notions concerning the elements (earth, air, fire, water) as composing the animal body, his therapeutic agencies consisted of a few drugs, steam baths, and injections.

Thomson's drugs were arranged mostly in six classes and known by number. For instance,

"No. 1" was emetic medicine, lobelia being his main drug for this purpose, which he used in enormous doses, and although there were repeated fatal causes of poisoning by the drug and numerous legal trials in consequence, "the Thomsonians insisted that lobelia was a perfectly harmless, innocuous medicine, not under any circumstances poisonous."

"No. 2" was stimulants—capsicum and the like.

"No. 3" consisted of astringents, or "canker medicine" and so on. This school was absorbed by the Eclectic school at Syracuse, New York, in 1843.

The Physio-Medicalis, which arose among the botanies about 1840 as an element of Thomsonianism is the only form which continues in existence in America, to any extent at least, at the present time.

In giving the history and progress of Drugless Therapy it goes back over an extended period.

The Aryans were the first to use this form of treatment, 3000 years B.C. also the Chinese in a crudely-developed form through a book called "Kong Fu" issued more than 20 centuries B.C. The Ancient Greeks and Romans, eminent physicians, used drugless treatment for its valuable therapeutic effects. The Japanese have practiced Drugless Therapy from immemorial times, and it has been in use by the Hindus and other oriental races since a remote antiquity. Its origin doubtless antedates that of the most ancient civilization of which we have records. The savage ancestors of those races practiced Drugless Therapy in some such primitive form as has been and is yet employed in Lomi-lomi of the Hawaiians, the Toogi-toogi, the Mili and Tota of the Tonga Islands, and in similar crude manipulations used by our own Navajo and Zuni Indians. Until early in the 19th century of our era, however, Drugless Therapy remained at best but a crude manipulation of the body, practiced without any adequate knowledge and without definite and intelligent method in its administration, and it had not yet been developed into a scientific method of healing. Peter Hendrick Ling through his untiring labors (1766-1837), a Swedish poet and physiologist that the world is indebted to for that very important advance in Drugless Therapy as now taught in the Royal Institution, founded by the Swedish Government at Stockholm, in 1813 and of which Ling was the first director. In this Institution, Drugless Therapy was for the first time placed upon a rational basis, was practiced in accordance with the anatomical and physiological knowledge of that day, and took its place in the recognition of leading continental physicians as an important agency in the healing art.

Massage was employed in some form by the Ancient Greeks and Romans, and by the Chinese, Japanese, Turks, Egyptians, Russians, and other races from the earliest times. Hippocrates, the father of medicine, says, "Anatripsis, a medicine applied by rubbing, can bind and loosen, can make flesh and rubbing causes parts to waste. Hard rubbing binds, soft rubbing makes them grow."

"Not only Hippocrates, but all the physicians and philosophers of that period, knew no better means of strengthening the vital principle and prolonging life than by moderation; the use of free and pure air, bathing, and, above all, by daily friction of the body, and exercise. The title given to this form of friction and exercise was **Gymnastics**, and was divided into athletic, military, and medical.

Herodicus, of Selivria, first proposed gymnastics for the cure of disease; and to such extent we are told, did he carry his ideas, that he compelled his patients to exercise and suffer their bodies to be rubbed; and he had the good fortune to lengthen for several years, by this method, the lives of so many enfeebled persons, that Plato reproached him for prolonging that existence of which they would have less and less enjoyment. Records show that some form of massage was used from the earliest stages of life. Some records dating back 3000 B.C. Martial (100 A.D.) Pling (102 A. D.) Galen (170 A.D.) up to Ling (1766-1837 A.D.) all recommended and used massage. From the ancient time until the present time the mode of rules governing massage have been greatly changed.

Dr. Mezger, of Amsterdam, about 1873, and Dr. S. Weir Mitchell, of Philadelphia, in 1877, improved and advanced the art of massage, and at the present day it is a well-recognized form of physical therapeutics.

"Ostrom," in his book on massage and Swedish movements (1902), writes that Mezger and his two pupils, the Swedish physicians "Berghman" and "Helleday" were among the first to apply the massage treatment in a scientific manner, the "Mezger" method being now used throughout Europe. He defines Swedish movements as a series of systematic exercises therapeutically applied to the human body, and then adds "Ling's" definition, "Every exercise, the direction and the duration of which are fixed, is a movement." Further, Ling gave every movement a double name, the first indicating the **position** of the patient; the second part telling the nature or kind of **movement**; as 1. **sitting,** 2. **rotation of the arms.** There are five principle positions in Ling's system; 1. Standing; 2. Sitting; 3 Lying; 4. Kneeling; 5. Suspending. From each one of these Ling formed many subdivisions of positions.

The movements are divided into two classes; 1. Single, which are subdivided into **active and passive;** 2. Double, sub-divided into **concentric and eccentric.**

The various movements also included; 1. Rotation. 2. Flexion and extension. 3. Separation and closing. 4. Bending. 5. Raising. 6. Pulling. 7. Turning. 8. Depression and Elevation.

An Open Letter By Dr. B. Lust To The Drugless Profession Of The United States Of America

by Benedict Lust

Herald of Health and the Naturopath, XXI (7). (1916)

Fellow Practitioners and Friends:

I take the opportunity to address you through this prospectus of the forthcoming Universal Naturopathic Directory, Year Book of Drugless Healing and Buyers' Guide. At heart I feel as though I should address to you a personal letter, but I would have to write 28,000 and that is not possible at present. What I would say to you in a private letter I can also say to you in an open letter—and here is the opportunity to reach you all without expense to the American Naturopathic Association on a large scale.

What is uppermost in my heart at the moment I dictate this letter is the American Naturopathic Association. You need this Association and the Association needs you. A new dispensation is being ushered in at this moment. We are living in a great time. Events take place and changes and reformation set in, for which it took formerly a generation to even prepare. History is being enacted. We are a part of history and we have to do our share for our cause, the noble profession of Drugless Healing which we represent, for our generation and generations to come. It is not by mere chance that we are Drugless Doctors. Sad experience, disappointment, the incompetency of the old school of medicine have forced us practically into the Drugless or Naturopathic Field. We all stand for the best and highest there is in the Rational and Progressive Healing Art. Our banner stands for exact science, for the shortest and best way to cure, for prevention of disease, life conservation along natural lines, through natural living, common sense hygiene, and we are solely and always guided by our unerring and infallible authority, Nature's laws. Our mission is to do good to our fellow men and to deliver the American people from the clutches and general exploitation of the Medical Trust; of those who are the slaves of this Trust, such as other medical schools who have sold their birthright, like the Homeopaths, the Eclectics—and the one drugless school, the Osteopaths, who have also sold their identity to the soulless idol and false god. By worshipping a false god you can never get to heaven. Shall we Naturopaths, Drugless Doctors of all schools and systems, also sell our birthright, go down on our knees and be governed, ruled, robbed of our individuality by these false gods?

For twenty years we have looked on; we have expected help from the Legislatures, the Federal Government, the administration of the cities in which we live, from the common sense of the American people and nothing good has been done for us. Persecution, jail, heavy fines, ridicule, condemnation by the subsidized press have been our lot. We have existed as sheep without a shepherd, without protection, without a standing before the law. Some of us have served prison sentences; some have lost their institutions and practice through unjust prosecutions; discriminated against and robbed of our civil rights. We have waited for years for leaders to come up, who would organize us, who would bring us together into one union, into one unit for progress, standardization, elevation of schools and for advance. Personally I have made a number of efforts. I toured the country last year and we succeeded in some instances in bringing about organization and consolidation of existing societies, but our efforts were not entirely successful; no constructive policy could be adopted; no practical results could be obtained; and all for one reason: Sectarianism, narrow-mindedness, lack of loyalty. It is immaterial to what school you belong, what system you practice; what light guides you; what you are—you need help and assistance for the protection and enforcement of your constitutional rights; for the breaking of unconstitutional laws; for the upholding of your constitutional rights before the courts, the press and society.

Do you believe, after an experience of twenty years, that things will change in the future; that you will come within your rights as a citizen, as a professional man, as a humanitarian, as an educator of the people in the art of natural living and prevention of disease, if you do not act yourself? No, you will go from bad to worse. Sooner or later you will find a loop thrown around your neck, from which is no escape. What is in store for you is the forfeiture of the little rights you have; the ostracism in your community; and the prospects of failure in life; unless you are protected and brought within your legitimate rights by a combination of the forces that are inherent in all of us.

In union is strength; in union we can break all the unconstitutional laws on the statute books in every state of the union; in union we can enact legislation that brings everyone within his rights; in union we can refuse submission to a mixed medical and osteopathic board, from whom we have never received a square deal in the past, now, nor get it in the future; in union we can demand recognition for our schools and for our successful practice; in union we can carry the legislature, the city council, the Board of Education; in union we can demand representation on the Board of Health in every State and city, in the health matters in the Federal Administration; in union you can kill every medical bill that discriminates against your constitutional rights; in union you can have splendid colleges, institutions and you can implant the principles of natural living and rational cure, of life conservation and efficiency in the school children, in the family, in the home and in all the public and charitable institutions; in union you can change the sad condition of affairs and break the grip of the medical trust and bring the American people to that great goal that is Health, Happiness and Efficiency; and in union you can prepare the road for natural living and Golden Age of peace, and the solution of every social question will be realized if everybody returns to the principles of Naturopathy, which means natural life, simple life and success in your chosen vocation.

Now, you will have through the American Naturopathic Association, representation and defense when you go into court. You will have a local, State as well as a National Lawyer at your disposal. Your fines can be paid and your case can be appealed. In every State of the Union cases can be brought to the highest court and if you don't get your rights the Association will carry your case to the Federal courts. The Association will advertise you and help you to establish a practice in your community. You will be listed in the different departments of the

Universal Naturopathic Directory every year. The official organ of the society will give you a continuous post-graduate course in the principle branches of Drugless Therapy. You will come in touch with the leaders, original thinkers and best of men in our profession.

The American Naturopathic Association is not a family affair; not a one man's affair. It is an association which is made up of seventeen State Societies, six of them having their own State Charters and at the yearly convention the delegates of the different State Associations elect their officers for the National Organization. A full financial and general account of the work of the Association is given at the yearly convention and in the official organ, the *Herald of Health and Naturopath*, you are kept posted of what is going on in the Drugless Field.

The Association will encourage all legitimate Drugless Colleges that stand for one or more branches of Drugless Healing. It will classify and standardize the schools and practitioners and it will in time weed out all the fake colleges and pretenders in the profession. Our Association stands for the best there is in the profession; for men and women of character and will act only in line with Drugless Therapy. We will preserve its identity, perfect it and built it up into one big whole in the only one and true science of healing, the Natural Drugless Art of Therapy.

Are you with us, or are you not? I appeal to you as a fellow practitioner and pioneer. I speak from experience, having gone through the different stages of a drugless doctor for the last twenty-five years.

The dues we ask of you are not high. They are a trifle compared with the benefits that will accrue. The initiation fee is $5.00 in States where there is no State or local organization as yet. This covers the first year's membership fees and you will get the official organ and full benefits. The yearly dues of the National Association are $3.00. Where, however, State Organizations exist the initiation fee is $10.00 and the yearly dues $5.00. For that the practitioner will have a Society behind him that works for legislation, protection, defense and every member will have the benefit of the Local and National Organization.

Kindly cut off the coupon at the end of this letter, forward with your fees and we will enroll you in the foremost and best Society for Drugless Therapy that there is in America. We are proud of our records. The Association has established seven schools, has raised the standard and efficiency in these, as well as in other colleges. It has delivered many a fellow practitioner from the clutches of the Medical Trust; has paid fines and lawyer's fees, and has succeeded in several instances in getting fellow members out of jail. The protective department of our Association alone should induce you to join the ranks of our members. Let us pull together for the common good, for legislation, protection and defense for the elevation of our profession, let us cast aside all prejudice on account of sectarianism or personal considerations and let us be guided by the higher ideals and the possibilities and future of the new school, the truly independent school, the Naturopathic or Drugless school.

All are welcome and you will never regret having backed up your school by a wall of strength and having become a true, solid link in the chain that embraces all that is good and rational in the healing art.

Yours for success and efficiency as Drugless practitioners,

B. LUST,
President, American Naturopathic Association

> *The Association has established seven schools, has raised the standard and efficiency in these, as well as in other colleges. It has delivered many a fellow practitioner from the clutches of the Medical Trust; has paid fines and lawyer's fees, and has succeeded in several instances in getting fellow members out of jail.*

1917

MEDICAL TYRANNY DEFIES THE CONSTITUTION OF THE UNITED STATES

BENEDICT LUST

———

EXTRACTS FROM LECTURE BY DR. WM. HAVARD AT THE N. Y. SCHOOL OF CHIROPRACTIC DURING THE 21ST ANNUAL CONVENTION OF THE A.N.A.

DR. W. E. HAVARD

THERE IS A CAUSE

Are you run down?
Tired out?
Nerves unsteady?
Do you feel shaky all over?
Are you weak?
Do you lack ambition and energy?
Do you have that "all gone" feeling when you get up in the morning?
Do you get up depressed, low-spirited, out of sorts?
Do you get exhausted and "played out" after very little effort?
Are you troubled with headache, neuralgia, pains in the joints and muscles?
Do you have dyspepsia, heartburn, belching, gas in the bowels, sour stomach?
Do you suffer from Rheumatism, Catarrh, Kidney trouble, Bilious attacks?
Are you subject to colds?
Have you lost hope of regaining your old time strength and health?
Do you know that all these ills come from one CAUSE?
Do you know that the only way to *permanently* rid yourself of these troubles is to eliminate the *cause?*
Don't take medicine. Medicines and drugs suppress symptoms, give relief, effect temporary "cures," but *cannot remove the cause* of the complaint.
Give Nature a chance, assist her in the right way, and Nature will surely cure you.
Your case is no worse—cannot be worse—than hundreds of others that have come to us and regained Health and Strength by our Natural Treatment without Drugs or Medicines. Do you wish to know THE CAUSE of your trouble and how to eliminate it?

Write today to

YUNGBORN HEALTH RESORT
BUTLER, N. J. AND TANGERINE, FLA.

Advertisement, October 1917, *Herald of Health and Naturopath*, XXII.

Medical Tyranny Defies The Constitution Of The United States

by Benedict Lust

Herald of Health and the Naturopath, XXII(4), 257-259. (1917).

The constitution of the United States guarantees the right of life, liberty and the pursuit of happiness to every citizen, but the vendors of official medicine regard the document which is the charter of our liberty, as simply a scrap of paper. The practice that prevails in the army of vaccinating soldiers with the poisonous pus of cow-pox, and inoculating them with typhoid vaccine, is a direct invasion, not only of the political rights of the soldier and sailor and airman, but is a deadly menace to the health of the person so inoculated.

What person in his right mind would drink the suppurating pus that oozes from the sores of cow-pox on the body of a calf? Yet to do so would not be one-tenth as dangerous as injecting such poisonous matter into the tissues of the body, because in the case of swallowing the poison, the digestive juices of the intestinal tract would probably disinfect and reduce to harmlessness such corruption, but in the case of direct transmission of decomposing material into the tissues, no antagonism from such digestive agents prevails, and the morbid matter is free to work with deadly effect.

What person, not an inmate of a madhouse would deliberately drink the poisonous juices boiled out of the bodies of dead typhoid microbes, the agents that allopaths assert are the cause of typhoid fever? And yet it would be a hundred times safer to do so than to inject such stuff into the helpless tissues direct, which is what is being done every time a soldier or sailor is being doped with this villainous vaccine.

Any army doctor will tell you that inoculation with typhoid vaccine is made compulsory in the American Army. In the year 1912, this compulsory edict went into effect. Yet the Surgeon-General in his medical report for this year states that there were 27 cases of typhoid fever of which there were four deaths. This left 23 recoveries of which, notwithstanding the statement that typhoid vaccination was absolutely compulsory in the army, sixteen of them, that is, two-thirds, **were not vaccinated.** The Surgeon General gives the history of why these sixteen were not vaccinated. Some were in Luzon fighting the Igorrotes, others were in Alaska, etc., but this whole bunch of unvaccinated soldiers completely disproved the oft-repeated assertion that typhoid vaccination is absolutely compulsory in the United States army. And this fact stares us in the face that all those who were not vaccinated recovered.

The Surgeon General goes on to say that the principal agent in suppressing typhoid is camp sanitation and rigid military hygiene. This he proves by pointing to the complete freedom from typhoid in the American Camps along the Mexican Border, but with regard to the condition of camp in which five thousand Mexican refugee soldiers, their wives and camp followers are interned, such is the ignorance regarding sanitation, such is the neglect of hygiene, that typhoid rages among them, in spite of the fact that every one of them was three times vaccinated.

Vaccination for small-pox is supposed to prevent that disease, but it is a well known fact that the majority of patients in the smallpox hospitals were once vaccinated. The vaccine virus left in the system through the inability of the organism to excrete it, manifests itself in many ways. It combines readily with any other disease, and awakens latent diseases. Pustular skin eruptions are very common and are often of deadly intensity. Many a fair face has been ruined by vaccination. The greasy, pimply, pustular, pitted skin of vaccination is indeed loathsome, and is carried through life. Lockjaw is a very common result of vaccination.

If these allopathic treatments are intended to preserve the health of soldiers, how is it we ask that the soldiers are so notoriously unhealthy? The personnel of both army and navy, not forgetting the aerial corps and the marines is composed of picked men from a physical standpoint, and only those are chosen who are free even from such slight defect as would not incapacitate them in a civil career.

In addition, these men are completely under the domination of the medical corps of the respective services, and must undergo such preventive, or remedial, measures as such medical superiors may see fit to prescribe. As to the essentials of life-food, shelter and clothing—the enlisted man is a far better position than the average citizen.

`With all this care bestowed upon him, it might be reasonably supposed that the enlisted man should be far healthier than the man who is compelled to shift for himself. But the contrary is true as the following official figures will testify:

In the ten years, from 1905 to 1914, inclusive, there was an annual average strength of the army of 69,741, while the total reported sick during such a period were 68,089, or 976 men reported sick for each 1000 enlisted. The days lost per case amounted to 13.58. During the period referred to, there were 3,657 deaths and 11,976 discharged on surgeons certificates of disability, or a total loss to the army of 15,583.

Now as to the navy and marine corps, statistics show that for the period under consideration, the enlisted strength mounted to 55,396, the average annual sick list amounted to 43,950, or 800 per 1,000 enlisted strength, while the days lost per case were 12.80. During the ten-year period there were 2,732 deaths and 14,125 discharged on surgeons certificates of disability, or a total loss of 16,587 men.

In the two services, every adult disease on the medical calendar was represented, including typhoid and small-pox, from which the men were supposed to be immune by vaccination.

Uniting the figures of both military and naval forces of the United States, we have a total average strength of 125,138 per year, for ten years, of which the total reported sick per year amounted to 112,040, or 888.38 per each 1,000 of enlisted strength, and the days lost per case were 13.19. For all the forces we have for ten years 6,389 deaths and 26,051 discharged on surgeons' certificates.

To appreciate the loss of these picked lives, let us say that if the army, navy and marine corps had remained stationary, with no enlistments, the loss from disease would have amounted to more than one fourth of the total force.

It may be claimed that this appalling death rate among our defenders was due to venereal disease. But it is a fact that the enlisted man is no worse off in this respect than his brother in civil life. The cause for the great amount of sickness and mortality in military life is due to the fact that medical masters of the men are encouraged in sowing disease in the individuals under their charge. Nature's bulwark against disease is rich red blood, uncontaminated by impurities. Befoul the purity of this precious stream, and consequences as dire as those described will surely follow, for when you once interfere with the order of nature, there is no knowing where the results will end.

It is the duty of the drugless practitioners to fight for medical freedom in the army and navy. Write to President Wilson and your Congressman letters of protest against the foul inoculations injected into the bodies of our soldiers, and sailors. Now that war is on, the poisoning of the life-blood of recruits will be carried on with increasing intensity. It is our duty to protect against the medical invasion of the rights of our brave defenders, who do not want their bodies infected with pustular poison of cow-pox or other equally poisonous serums and inoculations.

> *Any army doctor will tell you that inoculation with typhoid vaccine is made compulsory in the American Army. In the year 1912, this compulsory edict went into effect. Yet the Surgeon-General in his medical report for this year states that there were 27 cases of typhoid fever of which there were four deaths. This left 23 recoveries of which, notwithstanding the statement that typhoid vaccination was absolutely compulsory in the army, sixteen of them, that is, two-thirds,* **were not vaccinated.** *The Surgeon General gives the history of why these sixteen were not vaccinated. Some were in Luzon fighting the Igorrotes, others were in Alaska, etc., but this whole bunch of unvaccinated soldiers completely disproved the oft-repeated assertion that typhoid vaccination is absolutely compulsory in the United States army. And this fact stares us in the face that all those who were not vaccinated recovered.*

Extracts From Lecture By Dr. Wm. Havard At The N.Y. School Of Chiropractic During The 21ST Annual Convention Of The A.N.A.

by W. F. Havard, N.D.

Herald of Health and the Naturopath, **XXII**(6), 329-332. (1917)

Dr. Lust, I believe, struck a note in his talk just a few minutes ago to which we should give serious consideration, and that is the fact that women have entered politics. Don't overlook it. We have never received justice through man's politics, and wherever we have had men in **exclusive** control of anything, it has always led to corruption. (I might almost say the same thing regarding women). "Equal rights" will do much to solve the political question.

The reason that medicine has turned to brutality; the reason that it has sought for aggrandizement, is because it has been essentially a masculine institution. The women who have entered the profession are very few in comparison with the enormous number of men who have taken up this work, and of those who have, the majority fell by the wayside. We have always considered it a man's work; that medicine belonged to the male sex; that as a profession it would be degrading to women, and yet we never stopped to analyze our feelings or to determine why it degraded women. It could not be the profession itself—the healing of the sick that brought women students and practitioners down to the lower moral level. No; it was the awful contamination to which she was subjected in order to get her medical degree. Any of you who have been through a medical college, who have associated with medical students as a body, know what I am talking about, and any woman who comes through a medical college with a clean mind, must have had the support of all the angels in heaven. I might also say the same thing of hospital training for nurses; it is an abominable thing the way these things are conducted. The moral calibre of the medical profession, as a whole, is very low, and the only reason that our profession is better (and I know that it is, for it has higher ideals), is that we have freely admitted women to our institutions. Our women are the bulwark of the present drugless profession. The biggest part the men are doing is talking; the women are doing the work. Healing, as a profession, is really a woman's work. It requires that an individual possess a preponderance of the female propensities in order to inject into healing the necessary sympathy and all the higher qualities which are required of a physician. If Drugless Healing ever reaches its goal, it will be on the apron strings of the women. She will take it to the high places; but as she has always done since time immemorial. Just before we arrive, instead of dragging the men in, she will get behind and push them to the front. Men will get all the credit ultimately; but you can depend upon it that it will be the women who will carry the burden. Now, this isn't just for talk. I mean it. I really believe what I say; I really believe that the women are the power in this work; and just remember this fact, that before long, women are going to be the power in politics, and if you want what you want, and if you want it badly enough, approach the women; get it through them; don't bother with the men. You will never get anything from our present-day system of politics. You will never get the recognition that you are looking for under existing conditions; you will have to wait until women come in, and come in strong.

I believe women will clean out the hospitals, and put drugless practitioners in places of responsibility; but we will have to educate ourselves to assume these responsibilities, and that is what I am coming to. We are none of us any too sure of ourselves. I have heard people criticize Dr. Lee for his talk last night; but Dr. Lee has learned his lesson; he has tried everything, and he has found that nothing is **absolutely** reliable. That is a fact, no one thing in therapeutics will go the whole way; but we can find out the value of each thing and how far each will go toward effecting a cure. We are going after it in a systematic manner. We know now where we stand; we are on the road, but we are not too sure of the ultimate results we are going to get from the methods we are using. There are many improvements to be made, and much weeding out to be done. Very few of these newer systems have had the acid test. Many of our people have taken more or less short courses in various systems of healing, and do not know from their own experience the value of their methods. They only know what has been told them. Some are using them ignorantly, or by the chart or book. It requires the closest observation and a wealth of experience to master values; so we cannot expect the young men and women to have the same breadth of vision as those who have been in practice 20 or more years. We are none of us any too sure of our remedies, of the things we are using. We do not have it down to an exactness as yet. For one thing, we do not know human nature well enough. We have left this important study almost entirely out of our teachings. It is only recently that we have been teaching the characteristics of human nature. We have studied disease and cure, but not human nature. We must not only understand a person's physical condition, but understand how to approach that individual so we can know his capabilities and possibilities. This must be taught—the new doctor must be a philosopher as well.

Our crying need is a research institution; an institution where every graduate of any school whatever can come and build up his knowledge; where he can come and experiment, if necessary; where he can be turned loose in clinics under the direction of old, experienced practitioners, where he can gain confidence through actually seeing the things done.

We also need places, or at least a place, college or university, where the profession can send its sons, daughters and friends, knowing that they are going to be properly trained, properly handled, and that they will get the best of instruction. We not only need that for the profession, but we need an institution in which our children and children's children can be brought up in the ways of natural living. We need a kindergarten; we need a primary school, a high school, and a college, and ultimately we will need a university of Natural Life. Now you are educating the people daily; you are telling people this message; you are telling them that if a person is properly born and properly reared, there is no occasion to suffer disease; you are teaching natural methods of living; but you haven't the time to instruct all the people. The mother wants to know how to feed her children and how she is going to keep them from becoming diseased. Almost every day we have people coming to us, asking "What are we going to do, the Board of Health will not permit my child to attend school without vaccination?" They will not even take them at private schools unless they are vaccinated. We need schools for our children and for children of parents who want them properly instructed in the right way of preserving health. We want a school, not only for mental training, but of physical education, and of moral education. Naturopathy not only concerns itself with the physical welfare of the individual; it is a broad, liberal system, which teaches on all of the three planes—the physical, mental and moral. But what do they get in the public schools? Do your children get the right moral and physical training? No, they do not. They get largely mental training and that at too early an age.

We cannot confidently hope for the proper methods of training to be introduced in our public schools. We must establish our own institutions. It means a little sacrifice on the part of those who want to promote this sort of an institution. This is an ideal; something we desire to create; something we want to promote throughout this country, the world; but to begin we must establish one parent institution. It must be established. The schools we now have for teaching of Naturopathy are so limited that we cannot reach people we want to reach. It takes a group or body of individuals to devote themselves entirely to this work of organization. Dr. Lust has been too busy with work to do this thing alone. He has left this question to be decided by us, as to whether or not we are going to take the responsibility of starting and financing a college of Naturopathy, which college shall be the parent institution of all other institutions of its kind and character which shall be started throughout this country—the home of Naturopathy? We need not only schools and colleges to teach how to heal; not only training for doctors, but the training of the children from the cradle up. They are the kind of institutions to start. We want to teach people how to avoid disease. Remember that there are always people to practice on who will not listen to nature and reason; people who violate natural laws every day. Do not think when you begin to teach people how to live you will deprive yourself of bread and butter. You will not do that. As long as the medical profession is around the corner you will always have plenty of work to do.

Now, this is the question for us to decide, as to whether we want to start this movement for a national college, for a national university, and it is for you also to decide where this institution shall be located.

Now, I made a suggestion to Dr. Lust the other day. I said we ought to leave this matter to various state delegates to see how much money could be raised in different communities. The community that raised the most money would get the institution. Chicago wants it; Cleveland, Ohio, wants it. New Yorkers say they want it, but we haven't seen very much evidence as yet on the part of the New Yorkers.

Remember, it will not be for profit. It is not a money-making scheme. It will not be commercialized. It will have to be supported. It will have to be supported in the earlier stages by the profession itself. Do you want such an institution? Once you start it you will get endowments easy enough; but you must do the starting; you must show that you have at least the willingness to work for the furtherance of your ideals.

This must not be a "one-man" affair. A one-man institution in this work would never amount to anything; not on account of the man, but on account of the prejudice. People will not support an institution run by an individual, even though he is taking money out of his own pocket to run it.

We know that a college will not be self-supporting at first, and if you subscribe for stock in such a corporation or institution, you must not expect dividends for some time to come. It is immaterial to us if you do get money from wealthy patients; make an appeal to their sympathies.

We have to raise at least $25,000 to start this project, and we would be much better off to have $50,000, for you know if you make a good showing you get more consideration from students who come around to look at the institution. The stumbling block to greeting students into drugless schools is that they see nothing curious and wonderful to impress them. They have undoubtedly at some time been in a medical college, and seen the apparatus and equipment, and they naturally expect to see the same thing in a drugless school. Our school should have the right kind of equipment to make a favorable impression as well as for practical work.

Most of us do not come into this work intentionally; we stumble into it. It was by accident I entered; but it has a certain fascination,

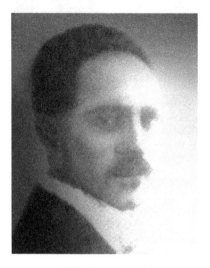

W. F. Havard, N.D.

and once you get into it, it ruins you for any other kind of work. You can't go back into business again because you are always preaching health to your business associates while they want to talk business. Once you get into this game you are absolutely ruined for business, so you might just as well make up your minds that in this, you must stick and see it through. Now, you can't go alone; you have to have some backing, and you might as well get the idea firmly planted in your minds. Ultimately, some time, we will all have to get together. No matter what our healing cult is, we must have a common institution behind us. Why not now? The barriers of sectarianism have been broken down, for here we are, graduates of all different kinds of schools, fraternizing on a common basis. The only thing that stands in our way is the money problem.

The plan which we wish to formulate now is to enlist the help of every one of our representatives in the field; as a matter of fact, of every member of the Association, and have them work a certain definite time, and work intensely to raise money by a certain date. This must not stretch out for years. We should have the money by a certain date; the trustees could then meet and decide where the institution will be erected.

Of course, we can't open the institution for this next term, but if we all get together and work, it will be an assured fact by next summer. Twenty-five thousand dollars isn't much to raise. Surely, among us all, we ought to be able to collect that amount of money by June 1, and by summer we could have all of our plans laid and even, possibly, the site of our location or institution decided on.

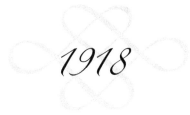

1918

1897   1918

TWENTY-SECOND

ANNUAL CONVENTION

of the

American Naturopathic Association

to be held at

Cleveland, Ohio

June 6th, 7th and 8th, 1918

Every State and local society should immediately elect their delegates.

Every Drugless Physician is welcome.

All Sessions open to the public. We have no secrets to withhold from the truth-seeker.

Everyone is invited to attend.

Delegates and members coming from a distance can have accommodations reserved for them by writing to the Convention Manager, Dr. Wm. Vernon Backus, Permanent Building, 746 Euclid Ave., Cleveland, O.

The American Naturopathic Association Annual Conventio attracted hundreds of delegates from around the world.

WHAT DOES THE A.N.A. MEAN TO YOU?

by W. F. Havard, N.D.

Herald of Health and the Naturopath, XXIII(4), 368-370. (1918)

This is a rambling talk, so have patience. It has a point, but some may miss it, so read carefully.

I wonder if you feel as I do about our organization. I wonder if you have the vision to see down the years to come? I wonder if you are preparing for the future? I wonder if you have an ideal in mind? Oh, I wonder so many things about you from day to day. Don't your ears burn? If you were in my place, I wonder what conclusion you would draw? If you had had your finger on the pulse of the movement as I have for a number of years, I wonder if you would feel discouraged? You would wonder too if you read all the letters that come in regarding the A.N.A You will not wonder, though, that I call some of you slackers if you'll but read to the end of this article. You'll know why.

Ask yourselves these questions:

Why am I in this work? Is it solely to make a living? Is Healing primarily a business with me? If it is, don't read any farther, for this article is not meant for you. Or do you feel that you are in this world, and particularly in this work, to make the world a better place to live in? Do you feel that you have a mission to perform besides feeding, clothing and housing yourself?

Do you get your joy and pleasure out of the consciousness of work well done?

Have you an ideal that you are striving to attain?

If so, you are the one to whom I want to talk. You will understand me. When you ask yourselves these questions, go before a mirror, look yourself squarely in the eye, and search your soul for an answer. Don't sidestep. I'm deadly in earnest. On your answer hangs the fate of this movement. Take it to yourself. Consider yourself the important factor in the work. Feel that the whole success depends on you and your effort. Labor as though you were the only one on whom responsibility

rested, and this movement will grow. If there are not a sufficient number of individuals willing to work in this way, there is no need of an
organization. Organization means organized effort for the fulfillment
of a purpose.

If we had only one hundred members, and if everyone felt his
personal responsibility, no power on earth could stop this movement.
We could laugh at the A. M. A. and their tools, the legislatures and
courts,—not forgetting the subsidized press. But suppose you did not
feel yourself an essential part of the machine, and you said "O, we've
got an organization to do the work, let the officers do the worrying,"
where do you suppose the movement would land? Your officers have
the spirit of philanthropists, but they are not millionaires. What are you
doing? Do you expect five dollars a year to bring "Kingdom Come"
to your door? Are you paying even that? Do you circulate the *Herald of Health* among your friends, patients, and acquaintances? Do
you solicit subscriptions for it? Don't feel that you would be putting
money in our pockets by so doing. If you sent in a thousand subscriptions it would not enrich us by one dollar. This magazine is dedicated
to the movement, and more money from this source would only mean
greater expansion and extension of your efforts; but at present, the publisher has the joy of paying all the bills. Your officers' hands are tied.
The movement cannot expand unless you help. We would like to see
the *Herald of Health* stand on its own feet before long.

Twenty years of pioneering in face of such obstacles would have
taken the heart out of a weaker man than our president. But, to
return. Whether you realize it or not, there is an organization to promote Naturopathy (the science and art of natural healing), The American Naturopathic Association, commonly called the A.N.A Now, what
does it mean to you? Why are you in it—if you are?

I'll tell you why some are **not** members (and this includes those who
consider themselves members, but who do not pay their dues or even
their magazine subscriptions). Because their minds are of such small
caliber that they cannot see beyond the immediate needs of the moment.
Because they have no faith in themselves and consequently can place

none in others. (Suppose a farmer had so little faith in himself and his soil that he would not sow his seed. Would he ever reap a harvest?) Their souls are shriveled up and their minds as impervious to an idea as a cocoanut shell. Some are not members because they are afraid that someone is making money on the movement. Why, the poor deluded hard-shells; how can they think such a thing? Even the undertaker will tell you that you can't make a living from drugless doctors. I will not mention names this time, but in a future issue we intend publishing a list of delinquent members. This is not a threat; it is exactly what is coming.

We want to know where you stand, so be quick to declare your intentions. We are going to weed out some deadwood. We are not telling you which flock we intend to keep. Sheep are useful for wool, but summer is coming and someone else always gets to them first and does the shearing anyway, so maybe we'll leave them to blat their troubles to the winds.

There is something in the air. Probably you have not sensed it yet. Things—big things—will begin to happen before long. It is up to you to determine whether or not you care to participate.

I'm talking to you as a fellow member of the A.N.A, not as an officer in the organization, and I'm talking this way because there are a goodly number of slackers in the association. Some of them are thoughtless. To them this is a reminder. Some of them are willing to take everything that comes along, but are too slack to pay the price. Those we don't want. We are not afraid of losing them. They are detrimental to the ideals and aims of the organization. We're glad to get rid of them. They are a hindrance to the movement. Lukewarmness is nauseating. Be one thing or the other. A fiery enemy is more valuable than a slack friend. To illustrate what I mean, I'll tell you a little story of a small man and what happened in Illinois last year.

When the new medical practice act was introduced into the legislature of that state, it looked very bad for those drugless practitioners who were licensed prior to July 1st, 1917, as it provided that they should all apply for new licenses, which would be granted only to those holding diplomas from recognized schools. Now there were many practitioners who had never graduated from any school, and many more whose schools were sure not to be recognized. So some of us got together and went down to Springfield to see what could be done about it. On our first visit, there was one very much agitated person in our ranks who claimed to be making several thousand dollars a year out of his practice, and was fearful of losing it. He was one of the non-graduates, by the way. He did a lot of talking, and made promises of what he would do by way of contributing to the legislative fund if we succeeded in protecting his license.

What was done has already been recorded elsewhere. After chasing around begging interviews with senators (ruining automobiles in our haste), and spending about one month of valuable time, the bill was amended and the old licenses remained valid. All this work had cost money, and a few individuals had dug deep into their pockets to pay the bills on the expectation that each practitioner who benefited would do his share. Letters were written—letters that would bring tears to the eyes—but very few substantial answers came in. But what about Mr. Man and his promises? Somebody told us what to expect, but we didn't believe it. We even offered to take him into our association before we got his answer to our appeal, which we had to go after. Here it is: "Well, you see, I've made enough, and I don't expect to be in practice much over a year anyhow, and I had that length of time before applying for a new license so the protection won't do me any good; besides, I'm a little short of money, but you may hear from me in a short time." Did we hear from him? Well, we wouldn't have spent his dime then if he had sent it. It surely would have found a resting place in a nice big frame.

Now, do you see what I mean? They are the kind that are better out of the way. They fool their patients for a little while, but the better practitioners in their towns gradually force them into oblivion. They go back to their trades from which some alluring advertisement, promising easy money, had called them. We can say a little requiem over them— they all go in time. No one really need bother to exterminate them.

They do it most effectively themselves. In this work, as in all other fields, the law of the survival of the fittest holds good. A practitioner in this work must stand on his own merits, and his sense of justice and fair dealing.

In the A.N.A, there is a place for everyone who has the interests of humanity and of natural healing at heart and desires to do good work. For the idealist there is the lecture platform and the pen, for the seed must be sown and the ideas planted in the minds of the truth seekers. For the experienced practitioner there is the field of demonstration, for the truth must be proven and made manifest. His work consists also in educating the younger generation of practitioners and extending the helping hand to the over anxious beginner with counsel and advice.

For the one with talent for organizing, the possibilities for the exercise of that talent are unlimited. Every city, town and village should have a nature cure center and health club. Societies of laymen should be organized to promote the science of natural healing and living. Here is work for the business man.

Where do you fit?

Or are you looking for immediate benefits?

Do you think the association should be primarily for defensive and protective purposes to give legal protection and provide a safe port in a storm?

Personally, I approve of the aggressive, constructive work. We must first create a position for natural healing, and if that position is strong enough, it will be a defense in itself. Our work is with the people, not with legislatures; and every time the opposition attacks us, it adds growth and strength to our cause.

Come, now; tell us what the A.N.A means to you. Be frank about it. Say what you think. Tell us what you consider its most important function, and we will do our utmost to have your ideals realized. I am, to all those of good will,

Fraternally,

Wm. F. Havard, N.D.

GREAT PIONEERS

by Benedict Lust

Herald of Health and Naturopath, XXIII(5), 446-447. (1918)

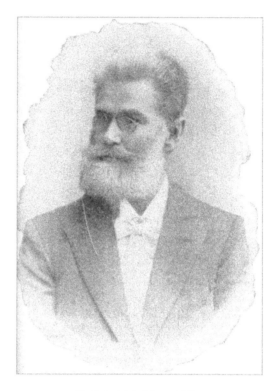

Dr. Friedrich Eduard Bilz.

That real physicians are born, not made, is well illustrated in the case of Dr. Bilz, who achieved his first success in healing as a lay practitioner. As a mark of gratitude, a wealthy patient presented him with land and a castle on which to found a Nature Cure Sanitarium. The medical profession apparently is not as watchful in Europe as it is in America, and wealthy patients possibly not so much concerned about leaving monuments to their names as they are interested in promoting good works. America suffers the disgrace of not having one wealthy patron of Natural Healing, while the state and Federal governments have actually hindered the advancement of the worthy science. They not only have refused a helping hand, but in most cases have turned a deaf ear to all supplications. The Bilz institution at Dresden-Radebeul, Germany, became world-renowned and was long considered the center of the Nature Cure movement. Prof. Bilz is the author of the first Naturopathic Encyclopaedia, *The Natural Method of Healing*, which has been translated into a dozen languages, and in German alone has run into one hundred and fifty editions. He has written many works on Nature Cure and Natural Life, among them being *The Future State*, in which he predicted the present world war, and advocated a Federation of Nations as the only logical solution of international problems.

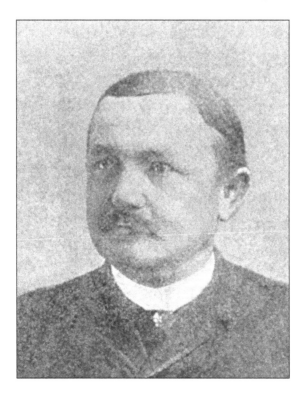

Dr. Katz.

As Surgeon-in-Chief of the Prussian Army during the Franco-Prussian war, Dr. Katz learned a thing or two regarding the treatment of wounds. He became convinced, through witnessing results, that antiseptics were more damaging than they were of benefit. (It has taken another war to prove this fact to a mentally dense and hide bound profession. A normal salt solution is now considered that best cleanser and dressing for wounds. Nature Cure has advocated this for many, many years.) Dr. Katz knowing at the time that it meant professional and social ostracism was big enough, broad enough to forsake convention and follow his convictions. He became a staunch advocate and practitioner of Natural Healing. He founded a Nature Cure Sanitarium at Hoehenwaldau-Degerloch, near Stuttgart, Germany, of which he continued as director until his death.

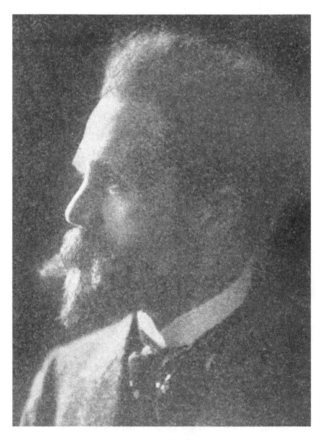

Dr. Henry Lahmann.

When the University of Leipzig expelled H. Lahmann for spreading medical sedition among the students, it added a staunch advocate to Natural Healing. Dr. Lahmann finished his medical education in Switzerland and returned to Germany to refute in practice the false ideas of medical science. He later founded the largest Nature Cure institution in the world at Weisser Hirsch, near Dresden, Saxony. He was a strong believer in the "Light and Air" cure and constructed the first appliances for the administration of electric light treatment and baths. He was the author of several books on Diet, Nature Cure and Heliotherapy. His works on diet are authoritative and his "nutritive salts theory" forms the basis of rational dietetic treatment. This work has but recently come to light in America and progressive dieticians are forsaking their old, worn-out, high protein, chemical and caloric theories for the "organic salts theory." Carque, Lindlahr, McCann, and other wide awake Food Scientists have adopted it as the basis of their work. Dr. Lahmann was a medical nihilist. He denounced medicine as unscientific and entirely experimental in its practice and lived to prove the saneness of his ideas as evidenced by his thousands of cured patients.

His works on diet are authoritative and his "nutritive salts theory" forms the basis of rational dietetic treatment. This work has but recently come to light in America and progressive dieticians are forsaking their old, worn-out, high protein, chemical and caloric theories for the "organic salts theory.

Dr. Lahmann was a medical nihilist. He denounced medicine as unscientific and entirely experimental in its practice and lived to prove the saneness of his ideas as evidenced by his thousands of cured patients.

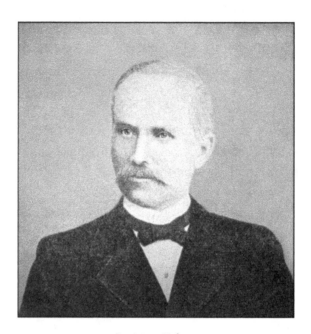

Dr. Louis Kuhne.

Louis Kuhne wrote, in 1861, the *New Science of Healing*, the greatest work of Basic Principles in rational Healing. His renowned work constitutes the only true Scientific Philosophy for the application of all Drugless Methods. He was the first to give to the world a comprehensible idea of pathology and the first to proclaim the doctrine of the "unity of disease" and the "unity of cure." His book "Facial Expression" gives the means of diagnosing a patient's pathological condition and determining the amount and location of the systemic encumbrance. He is the founder and first Master of Naturopathy.

Editorial: Our Schools And Colleges

by Benedict Lust

Herald of Health And Naturopath, XXIII(8), 709. (1918).

In little more than a month, a new college year will commence. The war has taken many and will take more of our able-bodied men who are now in, or about to enter, college. The number of male matriculants is very low, and many small schools and colleges – particularly those without endowment funds will be obliged to close their doors.

Plans have been made to carry out a big publicity campaign for Naturopathy. This, naturally, will create a big demand for naturopathic practitioners, but the work will be in vain unless we are in a position to supply the demand.

It behooves us, then, to see available men and women to enter Naturopathic colleges. An appeal should be made to men above the draft age and those exempt from draft, and, particularly, to women. Our profession is a most noble one, and women are most admirably suited for it. The woman is the natural healer. She possesses all the qualifications for the work, and more of her sex should be encouraged to take it up.

The objections that the sensitive, refined woman may raise to the study of medicine will not be found in the Naturopathic work. We are proud of the fact that our colleges maintain the highest standard of morality. The work and studies pursued in them are clean all the way through. Our institutions breathe an air of wholesomeness that strengthens the moral fibre of the student. No woman who has the natural aptitude for healing should overlook the opportunities which are offered in the Naturopathic field.

Help us fill our colleges, so that our noble calling may be well represented in the years to come.

SOCIAL HEALTH INSURANCE

Compulsory Health Insurance For Working People

by Benedict Lust

Herald of Health and Naturopath, XXIII(9), 761-762. (1918).

H OW will this measure affect drugless physicians?

There is not the slightest doubt but that if these measures now before several Legislatures are passed and become laws, it will bring the workingman more than ever under the autocratic control of the medical profession, for, although compulsory health insurance does not carry with it compulsory treatment, it goes without saying that the insured will be more likely to accept the medical benefits than if he were free to choose his favorite method of treatment. No one cares to pass up a benefit which he has already paid for. The drugless profession cannot, however, openly oppose these bills, except by showing the workingman the evils of them. For a complete discussion of social health insurance, we refer you to a series of articles beginning in the August first number of the *Truth Teller*. Space forbids us to enter into a discussion of the matter from the workingman's standpoint, which is purely an economical problem. But let us consider what would happen if social health insurance were instituted by law in every state, and medical and surgical attention forced upon the workingman. The workingman has felt the yoke of economic oppression and has arrived at the point where he will no longer submit to tyranny. He is now getting what he demands. He is no longer a wage slave. He is the backbone of industry, and, recognizing this, governments dare not set aside his just demands. Nothing would so quickly settle the question of whether we shall continue medical autocracy or whether we shall have freedom as for the medical profession to force measures upon the workingman and his family which he knows to be injurious. But how is he to know of the detrimental effects of medical and surgical treatment? What does he know about drugs, vaccine, serums and inoculations? At present, the average

workingman believes all medical treatment to be necessary and beneficial because he has never had the time or inclination to study and investigate. He bowed to the superior knowledge of the medical doctor because he knew of nothing else to depend upon in case of illness. There
was no choice, there was no question of choice; a doctor was a doctor,
and whatever he chose to do must be accepted as a matter of course.
The average workingman does not yet know that there are doctors and
doctors; he does not know that there is a medical question. Neither did
he know that, but a short time ago, he was imposed upon and abused,
overworked, underpaid and mistreated, until someone made him think,
and he began to realize that he was being squeezed by the capitalist
on the one hand, and milked dry by the profiteers on the other hand.
Not until he saw the cost of living rising out of all proportion to the
increase in wages; not until he realized that he was a slave to his work,
bound to the wheel, not daring to stop, because he and his family were
hardly more than three weeks removed from starvation; not until he
realized that such conditions would never be remedied until he made
his position known to the world; not until he saw the world indifferent
to his welfare, and not until he saw that his position was little understood did he take the only course left to him to effect an understanding.
He struck and showed the world how dependent it was upon his labors.
As a result of the awakened consciousness of the workingman, everything is done today to conciliate him. Governments are limbering their
stiff necks by bowing to him. Today, labor is king. It will fare ill with
the medical profession when the workingman realizes its autocratic grip
on the people.

STENOGRAPHIC REPORT

The Twenty-second Annual Convention of the American Naturopathic Association, held on June 6th, 7th, and 8th, 1918, at Hotel Winton, Cleveland, Ohio.

by W. F. Havard, N.D.

Herald of Health and Naturopath, XXIII(9), 764-767. (1918)

D r. William F. Havard gave an address on The Naturopathic Horizon as follows:

Mr. Chairman and gentleman: The subject is: "The Naturopathic Horizon." I would rather say, "The Naturopathic Situation As I See It." I don't expect everybody to agree with me. I have given up about eight months' time going around visiting the various centers, cities and communities where drugless practitioners are to be found, with the idea of sounding out the situation. I wanted to know what the various practitioners throughout the country thought. I wanted to find out what they were doing—what their ideas were—and their ideals were, if they had any—what they were looking forward to, and what they were really working for. I am not going to tell you all that I have found out, because it would not be fair. I am going to tell you my general impressions.

I found in some places that the practitioners were wholly and entirely selfish in practice and were conducting the practice purely for what it netted them in material gain. In other words, their practice was essentially a business proposition. They had no ideals. Their schools had taught them only the **business** of healing. They weren't working toward any end—except to put money in their pockets. This condition would be all right were the practice of drugless healing well established, if it were not for the fact that we are still pioneers; that we are still working to establish something; that we are still trying to place our practice—or our business, if you wish to call it that—on a firm foundation. If you will look back over our history and follow out the lines of development of our country, you will find that those individuals who forged ahead, who pushed westward, had to sacrifice something; they couldn't think entirely of material gains. They may have had that in the back of their minds. Their driving, compelling motive may have been individual, personal gain, either materially or by gaining greater freedom, but at the same time were sacrificing in many instances their lives for the purpose of developing the country. Now, I anticipate a probable question, and I acknowledge that behind everything there must be a selfish motive. We must all, every one of us, individually ask ourselves, before we enter into any special line of endeavor: what is there in it for me? What am I going to get out of it? This is necessary; we do not deny anyone that right. But besides that we feel that everyone should enter into the work that he is doing, not only with the idea of personal gain, but with the idea of establishing something which will be of inestimable benefit to those of his own period or to those who are to come after him. In other words, that he shall leave something behind him when he departs, which those who are left can look upon and say that it is good; that he did something; that he created something; that he accomplished a purpose, and in accomplishing that purpose that he has made conditions easier for those who followed him.

In other places that I have visited I have found individuals with these ideas, or ideals, if you choose to call them such. A great many of us fight shy of individuals with ideals; we think they are cranks. But let me tell you if it were not for individuals with imagination, with ideals, with the creative sense, if it were not for them cranks, the world would not progress. If you think that if all of the people who are satisfied with things as they are were to be given absolute control of the world's affairs that anything would move forward, you are very much mistaken. There would be no progress. There would be nothing done; there would be nothing accomplished to lay a better foundation for the future. Every time that something new is proposed, we are up against all of the opposition which is offered by the powers that be, because those powers are the ones who are satisfied with conditions as they are, because those conditions are either filling their pockets, or filling their stomachs. They are getting out of their everyday existence everything that they ask for; everything that they crave for; everything that they want. They will oppose everything that is new; they will oppose any progress that is instituted, and yet remember that in every case, in every instance where progress has been made, it has been made by a small group of people—not the majority of the people by any means. If we were all Edisons, why, this earth would fly off on a tangent and possibly go to its own destruction. It would move too rapidly. We have to have a certain limit; we must have conservative people; they are the balance wheel to our very existence. But we don't want to have too much conservatism. But remember, it is always the small force—I can't say the small force, I should say the small group of people with the big force, the people with constructive ideas and the people who can look into the future, who in reality mould that future condition. It is the thoughts of the progressive people today that will create the future state. Now, what are your thoughts? What do you want? What are your desires? Do you want to do something? Are you satisfied merely with tinkering the patients that come to you? Patching the spine here and the head there? If so, you are only patching up the conditions as they are, you are not really making the world any better. You are treating effects, not causes. You are not working for any improved future state. You are not working toward the point where you can picture in your mind, or your imagination, a world free from disease, because practically all these conditions will repeat themselves, and the more counteraction you use, the more encouragement you give the disease condition. Hasn't it been true of medicine? It has been exactly the same thing. The more medicine we have had, the more disease we have had. Now, the more drugless healing we have employed from the same standpoint, the more disease we will have. You are not wiping it out. Now, this drugless situation, as I see it, needs a little bit of its own medicine applied to it—it needs to be punched up. Wherever you go you hear drugless doctors talking about what big practices they have and what wonderful cures they are making, but if you stay in these towns a little while you can't see the evidence of it, and I have come to the conclusion that it is largely in their minds. They are self-deluded; they are self-satisfied, because they are making more money than they had ever hoped for. They think that they have attained the pinnacle of existence, and because they can now ride in automobiles they pat themselves on the back and say what great men they are. But how are they looked upon in their localities? How have they improved the cause that they are fighting for—if they are fighting? Really, we can not afford such arrogance.

Now, I have found in every instance that they have overlooked their one best bet, and that is the education of the people. That is the thing that they have paid very little attention to. One reason for it is this: they are afraid that if they educate the people to the point where the people are able to take care of themselves that that finishes their practice. But in this, they are mistaken. As long as you have the medical man around the corner, you need never fear of working yourself out of business by educating your people, because that medical man around the corner is making more cases for you every day than you can take care of. He is making more chronics than you could ever cure in your lifetime; and as long as you have the medical practitioner right alongside of you, don't you ever fear that you will lack patients or that you will work yourself out of business—you never will. Not in this generation or in two or three generations to come. You are safe from the business standpoint, perfectly safe. And if you will recognize this one thing, that your best factor in your success is the education of the people with who you come in contact, this movement would spread like wild fire. You wouldn't be able to stop it.

For the last three years, I have been connected with a sanitarium in Chicago, or an institution that has two sanitariums, and which conducts a college. We hold public meetings, health culture lectures, where we dispense free of charge to the public, information which will help the individual to bring himself to a state of better health. Now, do we lose business by it? No, indeed, we have increased our institutions in the last three years over fifty per cent, just through this work. Why? Well, remember that you, as doctors, with all that you know, when you get sick can you cure yourselves? Don't you have to go around the corner and look for another practitioner to give you an adjustment, punch you up a little; give you a little treatment and attention? Of course you do, every one of you do it. You don't take care of yourselves when you are sick. And these individuals who come in to those lectures and hear the talks and who take up our systems of diet and who adopt all the various health measures that we give them can't grasp it all in a minute, and if they are sick they come to us for personal, individual advice, and as a result they come to us as patients, and before you know it they are going through the cure, they are taking a full course, and it may extend over six months. You will never lose anything by following the same method. And here is the situation as I see it: That our individual doctors are too limited in their mental perceptions, too limited; they can't—to use a homely expression—determine on which side their bread is buttered. Whatever organization we have had, we have formed into little closed corporations with the purpose of holding on to what we have. Now, you all know the Bible story of the "Buried Talents." I am not going to repeat it to you. It is just another illustration of the drugless situation today. You are burying your talents. You are not making them as productive as they could be made; you are not sowing seed; you are not making an investment for the future.

Now, what is the remedy? It is not always wise to leave things hanging in the air, and the remedy as I see it is this: That there has to be more public propaganda in every community. I don't care how small the town is, there should be held at regular intervals public lectures, public meetings, for the purpose of educating the people along natural healing lines. You never know—you never realize how much you know until you attempt to tell it to somebody else, and you never grow so wise, mentally and morally, as you do when you teach.

Your work is not essentially that of treating the patients that come into your office, or relieving them of their little aches and pains, or adjusting their spines, and so on. That is not your real work, it is only a side issue to your work. Your real work should be educational. Educate the people into better ways of living and thinking, so that the next generation as it comes along will start out without the handicap of disease and disease suggestion, so that in time we may have here a wholesome, healthful nation of people, because it is only with that foundation of a healthy body and a sound mind that we can hope to rise out of this false idea that we have, at present, regarding civilization. You know, we have no civilizations. This condition that we are existing under is not a civilized state at all. It is only a thin veneer. We are not civilized. Scratch the varnish off the average man and you still find the barbarian underneath. Why? It all goes back to the same thing—wrong thinking; wrong eating; wrong methods of living; all the way through, man has built up within his body such conditions as will not allow him to express his true nature; they have hampered his mental and moral development. We are concerned with health. Health is the foundation of an efficient, progressive life, and we would like to see this nation rise to a height of intellectual, moral and physical development that would surpass anything that has ever been known in history, and that, in reality, is our fervent prayer, and it should be the mission of the naturopathic movement, that this nation will in time stand out as the savior of all nations. I thank you. (Applause.)

> *As long as you have the medical man around the corner, you need never fear of working yourself out of business by educating your people, because that medical man around the corner is making more cases for you every day than you can take care of. He is making more chronics than you could ever cure in your lifetime; and as long as you have the medical practitioner right alongside of you, don't you ever fear that you will lack patients or that you will work yourself out of business—you never will.*

Editorial: Naturopathy And The Epidemic

by Benedict Lust

Herald of Health and Naturopath, XXIII(12), 917-918. (1918)

One demonstration is worth a million theories. While our allopathic friends were futilely trying to check the "flu" with gauze masks, antiseptics, Dover's Powders and abundant food, and were wasting precious time trying to develop another poisonous serum from germs taken from the corpses of "flu" victims, the Naturopaths were achieving unrivaled successes. The death rate from pneumonia and influenza under Naturopathic treatment during the recent epidemic has been less than one percent. How does this compare with the fourteen to twenty percent and even higher, under allopathic treatment? A medical hospital unit of two hundred, en-route from Camp Lewis to Camp Millis, lost twenty-six men—greater causalities than they would have suffered on the battlefield.

A Nature Cure Institution in Chicago has an absolutely clean record. There was not one single death among the many cases treated by its staff of doctors and nurses, either inside or outside the institution. The Homeopaths have also had wonderful success. The death rate from pneumonia and influenza under their treatment has been negligible. In spite of the facts and figures proving allopathic inefficiency, it is this school of medicine that, through political intrigue, has saddled itself upon our army and navy. O, wait until this war is over, and we can speak freely and truly without being accused of treasonable utterances, we will bring in a bill against allopathic medicine that will rival the bill of indemnities that the German Government will have to pay for its vast devastations.

THERE WAS NO NECESSITY FOR ANYONE TO DIE FROM INFLUENZA. Every such death can be attributed to neglect, carelessness or mal-treatment.

When we place the Naturopathic record side by side with the allopathic, the people who do not join in the movement to overthrow the autocratic power of allopathic medicine, are fools and deserve no sympathy.

If they continue to accept the domination of the medical trust, they will have to abide by the consequences. Suppose we should refuse to treat these wrecks—the results of medical mal-practice and their own folly—perhaps it would wake the other fools up. The bulk of Naturopathic practice is among those who are on their way to the undertaker. We get them to salvage after the medico and the surgeon have done their best (?). My god, it is almost beyond belief that people can continue to be so stupid and ignorant. Let us make another attempt to prove to the people, by actual figures compiled from cases handled during this recent epidemic, that allopathic medicine is a false doctrine and a menace to health.

In order to prepare a proper report to submit to the people and the authorities, we desire every Naturopathic physician to report to us his cases, stating the number of Influenza patients treated during the epidemic, the number that developed pneumonia, the treatment employed, and the number of deaths that occurred, if any.

The death rate from pneumonia and influenza under Naturopathic treatment during the recent epidemic has been less than one percent. How does this compare with the fourteen to twenty percent and even higher, under allopathic treatment?

THERE WAS NO NECESSITY FOR ANYONE TO DIE FROM INFLUENZA.

1919

SHALL WE HAVE MEDICAL FREEDOM?
BERNARR MACFADDEN

INTOLERANCE OF OFFICIAL MEDICINE
BENEDICT LUST

THE EVENT OF THE CONVENTION
W. F. HAVARD N.D.

For Medical Freedom

By WM. F. HAVARD

I BELIEVE in Medical Liberty because I believe in human nature. I have more confidence in the doctrine of self-determination than I have in the doctrine of paternalism.

I believe that man's intelligence can only be developed through exercise and I believe that man's moral fibre would be strengthened through the assumption of individual responsibility for human welfare.

I believe that as long as the people permit others to think for them, to prescribe for them and to govern them, they will continue to be mentally, morally and physically diseased.

I believe that if all remnants of autocracy and paternalism were removed from our laws, the people would return to more natural conditions.

I believe that if people were given greater freedom of selection they would come closer to selecting that which is right and best for them.

But when a small group of people dictate what the vast majority shall do or what shall be done to their bodies, the wobbly boundary line between democracy and tyranny has been crossed and the individual sense of selection is dulled.

Our liberty, our freedom, has been stolen while we slept anl it is time the American people reclaimed their rights.

Dr. Benjamin Rush, one of the signers of the Declaration of Independence, predicted the very condition of medical tyranny which we have today, unless a guarantee of medical liberty was written into the Constitution. He was a far-sighted man but his advice was rejected.

It is not yet too late. The Constitution has been amended on other occasions and until this is done let us not boast too loudly of our democracy, our liberty, our justice or our independence.

Havard, W.F. (1919). For Medical Freedom.
Herald of Health and Naturopath, XXIV(4), 164.

Shall We Have Medical Freedom?

by Bernarr Macfadden

Herald of Health and Naturopath, XXIV(7), 336-337. (1919)

We have religious freedom in this country; we have freedom of speech. But medical freedom we have not. Do you want the liberty to decide what kind of treatment you shall have when you are sick?

In view of the fact that a large proportion of the people have lost faith in the old-fashioned school of medical practice, it would appear that the present control of all governmental policies concerned with the health of the people by the representatives of allopathic medicine, is a pure usurpation of power without the consent of the people and without representing the wishes of the people.

Is it better to die under "regular" allopathic treatment than to recover under the care of the drugless practitioner?

At a time when the practice of medicine is ceasing to be the practice of medicine, that is to say, when the medical profession is rapidly abandoning drug medication and learning to depend for results upon natural curative agencies, why are those who have had special training in the knowledge and application of these forms of drugless therapy denied the privilege of practicing or using this knowledge and these methods? If you wish to employ a drugless practitioner, the law steps in and says: "No! You must be treated by a regular."

Fortunately, however, there is one State in the union, regarded by many as the most progressive of all, in which the fight for medical freedom has been won. The legislature of the State of Washington a few months ago passed a bill providing for practice by drugless physicians. A board of examiners for drugless practitioners has been created, and only those possessing certain qualifications are permitted to practice.

What has been accomplished in Washington should be accomplished in other states. Medical freedom must be nationalized. Nothing can prevent the increase of interest in drugless treatment throughout the entire country.

A physician writing in *The Medical Summary*, August, 1919, says: "We as physicians have got to do more for the sick than ever before, or else we will see the Drugless Healers grow and fatten on our failures. As physicians we have failed in our duty to the sick; we have failed to find a definite treatment for the diseases common to our country. As a result of this sad state of things, there are thirty-five millions people in the United States that depend upon some form of drugless healing when they are sick. Where will the medical profession be in ten years from now?

"It is said that the average mortality from disease in this country would not be over seven per cent, without any medical treatment. The mortality under the treatment of some physicians is twelve per cent. From this it will be seen that the public would be better off without them. If we, as physicians, are to be of any real benefit to the public, the mortality under our treatment must be below seven per cent."

One objection constantly raised against drugless practitioners is that they are sometimes ignorant. But this can be met by establishing a standard of education and compelling them to pass an examination supervised by a State Board: just as the M. D. is compelled to pass such an examination. Practitioners without standards of education and proficiency are not desired.

There are now various societies concerned with the promotion of different forms of drugless treatment, each one battling "on its own." These may not have anything in common. Christian Scientists, for instance, may have little sympathy with any other form of treatment. And yet all of these have one thing in common and that is the right of freedom under the law to practice their systems of treatment.

Why should there not, therefore, be a national organization including all independent schools, this organization being devoted to securing legal recognition and the blessings of medical freedom? The influence of this association should be brought to bear upon the great political parties to induce these parties to include the cause of medical freedom as a plank in their respective platforms, while pressure is continuously brought to bear upon all legislators, State and National, in this direction.

If such an association for the promotion of medical freedom can be formed, the Physical Culture Corporation will agree to donate one thousand dollars to start a working fund, provided each of the national organizations of the Homeopaths, Christian Scientists, Osteopaths, Chiropractors, Naturopaths, and all other nationally organized schools of healing opposed to Allopathic Medicine, will donate a similar sum to start an organization with the object of calling a National convention that will form plans for a political union of all forces against Allopathic domination, governmental and otherwise.

Dr. Cabot of Boston has said that there are only six drugs in the world that are effective in any case, and that nature given half a chance would complete the cure herself.

Why not give her the chance?

Let us hear from those interested.

—Bernarr Macfadden, Editor Physical Culture

Do you want the liberty to decide what kind of treatment you shall have when you are sick?

It is said that the average mortality from disease in this country would not be over seven per cent, without any medical treatment. The mortality under the treatment of some physicians is twelve percent.

INTOLERANCE OF OFFICIAL MEDICINE

by Benedict Lust

Herald of Health and Naturopath, XXIV(9), 438-440. (1919)

During this period of reconstruction for the establishment of true democracy and the furtherance of genuine humanity, we should not overlook the importance of bringing home to the American people that true welfare cannot exist for the people of the United States unless we have our educational and economic systems based on natural law, and that the people receive education and liberties which will safeguard their physical, mental, and moral health.

The foundation of all reform, human happiness, physical and mental efficiency and morals, has its roots in a rational, natural life.

The greatest obstacle we have to contend with at present is the obstinacy, the autocratic self-constituted control of the medical combine, in other words, the medical imposition as it has fastened itself upon the American people.

In every avenue of human endeavor we see to-day the secret, and in many instances, the open, working of the American Medical Trust, the A. M. A. In all the lawmaking bodies, federal, state, and municipal, in the boards of health, in the board of education, in the army and navy departments, their ruling power is supreme and the last word. They are exercising police power, which has never been given them by the people, for enforcing their unnatural health-undermining, disease-breeding, and slow-poisoning methods against the American people.

The world war has been terrible in its direct and indirect destruction of human life, but its destructive work is small as compared with the destruction of life through **medical** superstition and exploitation.

This medical oligarchy is branding as imposters and criminals everybody that does not submit to its self-constituted power, refuses recognition of everything that does not agree with its rulings.

I, as one who has suffered much from several operations, from six vaccinations enforced upon me in different parts of the world, with the result that I was finally stricken with consumption. When being down and out, 20 years old, and weighing only 104 pounds, having been given up to die, I finally found the Nature Cure, the great system of the famous Father Kneipp of Woerishofen, Bavaria. He put me under the environment and treatment that gave me back my health by drugless methods. This was the turning-point of my life. After I was saved from the brink of the grave, I studied Father Kneipp's methods and, became one of his pupils. In the year 1896, I was sent by him to America to introduce the Kneipp methods and I received at the same time a commission from the National Association of Drugless Physicians of Germany to transplant the Nature Cure movement to the United States. That I have done so successfully was acknowledged by the Kneipp Society of Germany and by the National Association of Drugless Physicians, and I received in the year 1899 a gold medal and an honorary diploma for distinguished services rendered to mankind. Much has been said and written, true and untrue, about autocracy in Germany, but so much is sure that in my instance I received an official recognition from the German Government for transplanting drugless methods to the United States. To me it seemed a very humane government, interested in the welfare of the people. But what did I receive here? From the very outset I was hounded and prosecuted by emissaries, sleuths, detectives, stool-pigeons, and spittle-lickers of the New York County Medical Association. I was arrested fourteen times for practicing the Nature Cure. In the year 1899, when the judges still were human and dismissed such cases and after my case was discharged by the judges in the Court of Special Sessions, my lawyer introduced me to the lawyer of the N.Y.C. Medical Society, with the following words: "I take pleasure in introducing Dr. Lust to you, who is not that kind of a man that you have in mind," and who replied: "I think Dr. Lust is an honest man, and is sincere about his Nature Cure work, but it is that Kneipp system and Nature Cure he represents that we are ordered to root out." The next time I was arrested because one of the sleuths took a bath and massage treatment in my water cure establishment, "for the practice of medicine and surgery without a license," I asked the judge to let me explain, and he said : "I am no authority to decide whether baths, massage, and exercise constitute the practice of medicine or not, but I put you under $600 bail and hold you for the special sessions," and then he asked me whether I had a lawyer and a bondsman. I said: "Your honor, I have committed no crime, I am a respectable citizen." But this was of no avail, I was thrown in the pen, and held until the next day when a bondsman could be procured. The case was finally tried and I lost it, being fined $200 for conducting a bath establishment, giving massage, exercise, and diet, and my assistant was also fined $200 for administering the bath and massage treatment. I paid under protest and one of the three judges said: "There is no evidence that you practiced medicine of surgery, or held yourself out as a physician, but we fine you all the same." $400 fine for me and my bath attendant, and $400 for lawyer fees, together $800. I declared in open court that each dollar spent for fine and lawyer fees must mean an additional drugless doctor. The medical society lawyer in making his final appeal to the court said: "As far as this man Benedict Lust is concerned, I ask your honor to give him in addition to a heavy fine a long prison sentence, as he is the leader of these drugless imposters, has established a society of the so-called Nature doctors, and advocates in his magazines and other publications the open violation of the medical law." Not satisfied with such treatment we kept on fighting and in the next issue of the Naturopath Magazine I published the full story of my trial and I was arrested afterwards for criminal libel for the following two sentences in that editorial: "A man or a woman who conducts a Nature Cure establishment, gives baths, massage and exercise is not committing a crime, the assistant or nurse who dispenses the bath and massage and exercise is not a criminal; but when the sleuth of the New York County Medical Society comes around, takes a bath a crime has been committed. Who was the criminal? In every drugless case where this woman sleuth figured (there were at that time 45 cases in New York City where drugless doctors received the same treatment I did) she was the criminal. She is a disgrace to American womanhood and to the free soil of America on which she trods." I was arrested and hand-cuffed in my office, and carried to the

Tombs as if I had committed a murder. I was put under $3,000 bail, later on indicted by the grand jury for criminal libel, and bail raised to $10,000. After being eighteen times in court, the case finally to be tried. My lawyers at that time demanded in open court that this association, the Medical Trust of New York City, show its character to the jury, so as to see whether it received from the New York Legislature ever such authorization as to exercise police power. What happened? They were not prepared, and the next day offered a retraction.

These are some of my experiences as a drugless doctor. In order to practice drugless methods in this State, I had to take up the study of medicine, in which I did not believe.

The drugless movement will eventually entirely replace official medicine, as it is the only rational method of healing that has a real natural basis as a healing art, the prevention of disease by natural life. Drugless colleges should be more encouraged by the public and legislation enacted to make the healing art free, to give us medical freedom, as the countries of the old world have it, always had it, even in autocratic Germany under the Kaiser and under the Czar in Russia. The American Medical Association is a curse to the American people, keeps the public in ignorance, has never imparted any real information to the people on the prevention of disease. Their measures are contrary to real progress in medicine. The art of healing is simple, and easily carried out by anyone who has common sense. Medical laws are all class laws and unconstitutional in their last analysis. The people should control through laws the dispensing of poisonous drugs, and doctors should be held responsible for what they do by the general penal code. Surgery and obstetrics should also be controlled, but no laws should be made that prohibit the prevention of disease by natural methods of living and healing or the practice of anyone of the drugless cults, such as Nature Cure, Physical Culture. Keeping fit physically, morally, and spiritually is the only true preventive of disease. Vaccination and all other compulsory measures of the Medical Trust as practiced to-day are contrary to all natural law, to all common sense. All old medical laws should be wiped off the books, and medical doctors in practice and those who are in medical schools now, everyone should pass an examination in drug-less methods, and each one should have to prove, first, whether he is physically and mentally fit to be entrusted with the health of the people, as at present most are not. Without free competition in the art of heal-ing, the American people will be deprived of their inalienable rights under the Constitution to select the method and the doctor of their choice and to have the best in the prevention and cure of disease.

In the new era of reconstruction, where the people will think for themselves, medical autocracy will have no more place and the drug-less healing and physical culture movement will come into its own. All the work of the American Medical Association for the prevention and cure of disease cannot compare with the constructive value for the real prevention and cure of disease of one issue of *The Herald of Health and Naturopath*.

This magazine will also champion in the future as in the past the case of natural life, physical culture, natural cure, chiropractic, clean and moral eating, and hasten the day when medical graft which is noth-ing more or less than a continuation of superstition, sorcery, and magic of antiquity will disappear forever. Only cleanliness and vitality prevent and cure disease.

Without free competition in the art of healing, the American people will be deprived of their inalienable rights under the Constitution to select the method and the doctor of their choice and to have the best in the prevention and cure of disease.

The Event Of The Convention

by W. F. Havard, N.D.

Herald of Health and Naturopath, XXIV(12), 583-584. (1919)

There never was such rejoicing in the land of naturopathy as reigned when Dr. E. R. Moras of Chicago, and Dr. Wm. George of Columbus responded so handsomely to the appeal of Dr. Alzamon Ira Lucas of Portland, Ore., for funds to found and erect the American Drugless University.

Over seven hundred physicians and followers of natural methods of healing filled the convention hall in the Hotel Commodore on November 6, 1919, when Dr. Lucas made his inspired speech and over seven hundred hearts went out to him in that hour. He instilled the spirit into the Convention that caused those who came as spectators to feel themselves an essential factor in the great work of letting light through the dark clouds of superstition that hover over the field of healing.

The foundation of the American Drugless University will insure the benefits of every valuable method of healing to future generations. Historians of the future in searching the past of naturopathy will recognize in the records of the Twenty-third Convention of the A.N.A the turning point in its progress.

For years Dr. Lust and his co-workers have labored to bring about an affiliation of interests that could make possible the establishment of a great parent institution representative of the best that has been evolved in the healing arts. The opportunity has been offered to many but they were without sufficient foresight to see the possibilities.

Dr. Lucas came at the psychological moment and brought to fruition the labors of Dr. Lust and the pioneers of naturopathy in America.

Does it not make your heart rejoice to know that our University will be? Are you not thankful for the splendid, unselfish generosity of such men as Dr. Moras and Dr. George? Should we not be eternally grateful to Dr. Lucas and should we not congratulate Dr. Lust on his success? Be it remembered that he is the one who had kept the altar fire burning through all these years of discouragement. He has never lost faith even in the darkest hours but has worked with single hearted purpose toward his objective.

But these men do not want thanks, gratitude or congratulations. They want your substantial support.

Five million dollars is needed to build and endow this university. The American Medical Association through its tool the Red Cross can raise a hundred million to medicate and serumize the American public. Can't we raise a fraction of this sum to do a greater work?

Think what such a university will mean! It will establish drugless healing in its rightful position at the very pinnacle of the arts and sciences that are conferring benefit upon humanity.

Here is your opportunity. Are you big enough to meet it? Do you want your name on the honor roll beside those who are willing to sacrifice their all for the realization of their ideals? Would you like to look into the future and see your children, your children's children and their children on down through the years point with pride to the mighty edifice that your energy, your work, and your money helped to erect?

Then give from the fullness of your generous heart that you may be remembered for what you have done.

This is a drugless healing's big day. The child of our dreams has grown to manhood. We must start him on the road to his greater success equipped with every requirement to meet the demands of an ever growing and increasingly intelligent world.

Every dollar you contribute and every subscription you secure will reflect back to you in success, prosperity and happiness.

WM. F. Havard, Secretary, A.N.A

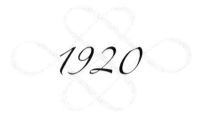

1920

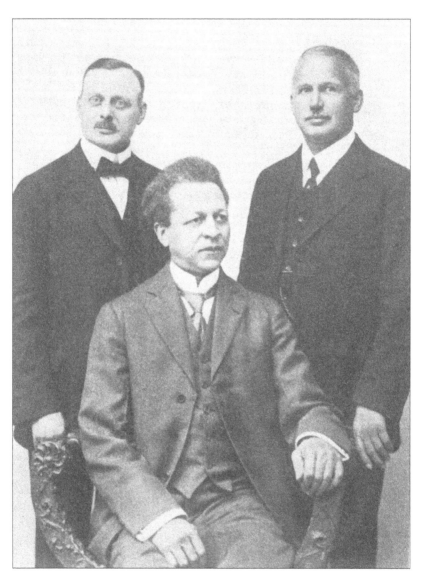

Dr. F. W. Collins, Candidate For the Presidency of the United States,
with his committee, Drs. A. I. Lucas and Benedict Lust,
Herald of Health and Naturopath, XXV(6).

WHO WILL GIVE THE FIRST MILLION TO PROMOTE NATUROPATHY?

by Benedict Lust

Herald of Health and Naturopath, XXV(2), 61-62. (1920).

We read with interest that "The Carnegie Corporation of New York has announced its purpose to give $5,000,000 for the use of the National Academy of Sciences and the National Research Council.......The council is a democratic organization based upon some forty of the great scientific and engineering societies of the country....... The council was organized in 1916 as a measure of national prepared-ness and its efforts during the war were mostly confined to assisting the government in the solution of pressing war-time problems involv-ing scientific investigation. Reorganized on a peace-time footing it is now attempting to stimulate and promote scientific research in agri-culture, medicine and industry, and in every field of pure science. The war afforded a convincing demonstration of the dependence of modern nations upon scientific achievement, and nothing is more certain than that the United States will ultimately fall behind in its competition with the other great peoples of the world unless there be persistent and energetic effort expended to foster scientific research". We realize that, of all the sciences, medicine is possibly the most backward and so does everybody else, consequently it is more than likely that the National Research Council will devote most of its time and the greater part of this endowment in chasing new "bugs" and inventing new serums. It is a lamentable fact that the surplus fortunes of our great millionaires are being poured into the coffers of a parasitic institution to promote the most gigantic hoax of modern times—the germ theory. If it were a hoax that merely wasted time and money we might enjoy the joke, laugh and forget about it; but it is becoming such a serious menace to our lives and happiness that anyone with a spark of feeling in his body cannot help resenting the vicious propaganda of medical organizations and so-called research institutions, which is driving or persuading the people to pollute their bodies with bacterial products in the name of prophylaxis.

We who know the law and who realize that acute diseases are cleansing processes, can see that by suppressing one such process we only lay the foundation for a more severe reaction. We know that all foreign matter that enters the blood must be neutralized, oxidized and removed by the eliminating organs and when the task is too great for the organs to accomplish by ordinary means, a reaction sets in. This is called an acute disease. It is these acute conditions that serum and vaccine therapy have been endeavoring to suppress. But Nature cannot be outwitted. She is always one or two jumps ahead of the latest attempts to thwart her constructive efforts. About the time that "science" rubs its hands and says, "Now we have the means of controlling every dangerous (?) acute disease", a new disease develops or an old one appears in a slightly changed form and the great science of medicine is compelled to acknowledge its helplessness. In any semi-civilized country it is certain that the "medicine men" would be asked for an explanation and would be held accountable for such an occurrence as the "flu disaster", but we let our medical dictators get away with a lame excuse. Modern medical research means looking for bugs and preparing serums, vaccines and antitoxins. Money spent for such purposes would be better thrown to the dogs.

Suppose someone should give us an endowment of $5,000,000 to promote and popularize NATURAL HEALING and HYGIENIC LIVING, think of the great amount of real good we could do. Think of how far we could carry our message with even half that sum when you consider what has already been done without a fund of any sort.

FACING THE SITUATION

by Benedict Lust

Herald of Health and Naturopath, XXV(6), 269, 283. (1920).

Naturopathic leaders have long cherished a fond dream—the union of all drugless factions into one great profession. Now they must acknowledge that it was only a dream. It looked feasible, it seemed reasonable considering that the factions had so much in common. Naturopaths have neglected their own work, have sacrificed opportunity after opportunity to push their own ideas to the front, in endeavoring to promote the greater union.

Now we must look the situation squarely in the face, give up our dreaming and settle down to work. Let the Osteopaths, the Chiropractors, the Mental Therapists and all the rest of the one-track systems go their own separate, independent ways. Let honest competition and the growing intelligence of the public relegate each to its proper sphere.

We have dwelt so long on the idea of union that Naturopathy has come to be looked upon as a hodge-podge of drugless methods of healing. While it is true that Naturopathy has absorbed all that is valuable in manual, mechanical, mental and other systems of therapeutics, it existed long before any of these newer systems were invented. Its growth has been slow due to the fact that it places the blame for disease where it belongs—on the ignorance of the people or their willful disobedience of natural law. It likewise places the responsibility for cure on the individual. For this reason it cannot be very popular among a people who dislike to be told plain truths. The educated as well as the uneducated eagerly grasp at any idea, no matter how illogical, that will place the blame on some thing, condition or circumstance over which they have no control, hence the germ theory, the bony lesion and subluxation theories have become vogue.

Naturopathy has actually compromised its position by encouraging the growth of these various systems. It has led to the assumption that Naturopaths agree with the theories of these schools. As a matter of fact a real Naturopath could not subscribe to the Chiropractic theory of disease causation. He might adopt chiropractic treatment as a means of assisting in the clearing up of disease **effects** but he could never fool himself that he were treating the **cause** by such a method.

Chiropractic, Osteopathy and all other systems have their places and they are supplying a demand. People are still ignorant of their bodies and the way they should be cared for. It is the tendency of the age to cover up effects and overlook the cause. When you desire to enter business it is much easier to determine what the people want and then sell it to them than to educate them to what is best for them.

Nevertheless the latter is the field of the Naturopath. He is essentially an educator. If he looks upon his work as a commercial business he had better get into some other field for he cannot remain true to his calling when he finds that more money can be more easily made by supplying the popular demand for palliatives.

Let the factions fight their little fight for supremacy. It will eventually bring out the truth. The time has come when we must attend to our own knitting. We have a message to deliver but we have been so busy trying to unite uncongenial elements that we have forgotten our real work. Let us settle down to it now.

Naturopathic principles are unassailable. They are based on natural law. It is unnecessary to defend them. But they do require to be taught and expounded to those who never heard of natural law.

The crying need of the naturopathic work is more propaganda for natural living and healing and less compromise with superficial methods of treatment.

Treatments of all sorts may be what the people want but what they need is a knowledge of the principles of right living. Keeping people well is a greater art and a more magnificent work than peddling treatments.

The time will come before long when the people will demand the services of the physician who can keep them well and teach them how to live and the one who merely patches up the sick person so that he can perpetuate his misery will be a back number.

The true naturopath knows the science and art of health. He is a health expert and as such he has a monopoly of the field.

The course of duty lies plainly before us. Let us not again be side-tracked from our purpose.

Let the factions fight their little fight for supremacy. It will eventually bring out the truth. The time has come when we must attend to our own knitting. We have a message to deliver but we have been so busy trying to unite uncongenial elements that we have forgotten our real work. Let us settle down to it now.

Naturopathic principles are unassailable. They are based on natural law. It is unnecessary to defend them. But they do require to be taught and expounded to those who never heard of natural law.

The crying need of the naturopathic work is more propaganda for natural living and healing and less compromise with superficial methods of treatment.

EDITORIALS: A NEW USE FOR THE INJUNCTION

by Benedict Lust

Herald of Health and Naturopath, XXIV(7), 321-322. (1920)

The medical profession of Illinois has brought a new weapon with which to fight unlicensed drugless practitioners. Injunctions have been secured against fifty or more Chiropractors to prevent them from taking advantage of the protection offered by their Association. They dare not pay dues into the organization nor accept money of legal aid from the Association for fear of arrest for violation of the Illinois Medical Practice Act.

The success of the Government's injunctions against the striking miners and steel workers evidently suggested this procedure to the medical organization. The cases are not parallel, however. Strikes disturb the economic situation of the country and work a hardship upon the people as a whole, whereas the practice of drugless healing is a benefit to all but the medical profession. Here we have injunctions being used to eliminate competition, the injunction suits actually being brought by a department of State government – the Department of Education and Registration.

What a deplorable situation when an individual who believes he is doing what he has a moral right to do can be robbed at the start of his greatest means of defense.

All that we can say is that the medical profession is desperate. The plan was laid early in 1917 to eliminate the Chiropractor as a business competitor. Early in that year the Medics and Osteopaths of Illinois schemed to rob the already licensed drugless practitioners of the right to practice their respective arts obtained under the then existing Practice Act which was adequate and sufficient to meet all the demands. The bill they presented to the legislature was so amended as to protect those already licensed but raised the qualifications immediately to such a high standard that only one or two osteopathic colleges could meet them. No chiropractor can now obtain a license. That it was the intention of the framers of the bill to discriminate against all but osteopaths and medics is proven by the fact that the requirements for drugless practitioners were fixed at the highest osteopathic standard which they had only attained after over thirty years of effort, and in raising the medical requirements they gave all students then in colleges an opportunity to finish under the old requirements. But no conclusion was given to any other profession. Class legislation with a vengeance.

Is it any wonder that Chiropractors and Naturopaths ignored this law? The medical profession forgets that it is but a few years since a medical degree could be obtained in two short years. The osteopathic profession forgets that but a few years ago osteopaths were made in one year and we defy anyone to say that the present brand of medical ape being turned out of a four-year osteopathic course is any better product, can bring any more benefit to suffering humanity than our old A. T. Still. Osteopaths who finished their courses in one and two years. Professions require to be built, they are not hand made. Legislatures should encourage infant professions instead of being the tool of trust-like competitors who desire their extermination for their own profit.

The consequence of this colossal piece of injustice has been to flood Illinois with unlicensed practitioners.

Panic has seized upon the medical and osteopathic organizations. Now they are out to kill. But so far prosecution has been a failure, the number of convictions under the new law being almost negligible. Cases have been continued until forgotten. Those which came to trial and were lost by the defendants have been carried to higher courts. Some have been thrown out of court on technicalities. The time of the courts is being wasted and the people's good money being spent in vainly trying to protect the old against the new. The new will ultimately triumph. It is in the nature of things. But in the meantime we shall witness a glorious battle. The attacking party has won the first skirmish and has robbed the defense of some of its weapons. What will the chiropractors do?

We hope they are intelligent enough to see their way around these injunctions. There is a big flaw in the present law and if the chiropractors can find it they can enjoin the Department of Registration and Education from further action until this point is settled. The law regulating the practice of Optometry in Illinois was declared null and void a few years ago because it contained the same mistakes as the present Medical Practice Act. No case as yet had been defended on this ground. A law which shows favoritism toward any class is unjust and this law has at least two instances of this type of injustice. Let the law sharks get busy.

THINGS FOR CONSIDERATION AT THE CONVENTION

by Benedict Lust

Herald of Health and Naturopath, XXV(8), 373-374. (1920)

The American Naturopathic Association has tried to play god-father to every system and method of drugless therapy that recent times have brought forth. We have now come to the point where we see that these precocious youngsters are more than able to take care of themselves. They no longer desire the help which we might be able to extend to them. They are determined to go their own separate, individual ways as children of this age are prone to do, waging their own battles and standing or falling according to their merits. It is necessary then that the A.N.A adopt some definite policy in dealing with other associations representing practitioners of different methods of drugless therapy and with individuals of these schools.

Instead of one family of individuals each of which may hold slightly different opinions, the drugless movement is divided into factions which have become estranged from one another and a number of bitter feuds have been engendered which are likely to retard rather than further the interests of the different factions.

This convention should go on record as a mediator of disputes and should outline a policy of co-operation on the broader issues to which all could adhere without detracting in any measure from the individuality of any system.

Heretofore it has been our policy to admit any practitioner of or believer in any form of drugless practice without first determining whether or not that individual understood the fundamental principles of naturopathy, consequently we have in our ranks many who are unable to further the cause on account of their limitations. These people are well intentioned but very often spread misinformation regarding naturopathy. The second consideration for the coming convention is to determine what qualifications a naturopath should possess and to make such qualifications necessary to admission to active membership into the association.

The third consideration is to devise ways and means of firmly implanting the principles of naturopathy in the minds of the drugless practitioners. To a certain extent this means free education and every true blue naturopath should be impressed into service in this cause.

The fourth consideration is that of wider publicity for our principles and methods. A committee on publicity should be appointed which would furnish subject matter for magazine articles, letters to newspapers, tracts, etc. The first thing to be devised is a catechism for naturopaths. This sounds rather orthodox but a series of questions and answers is one of the best means of impressing principles and fundamentals upon the mind.

A thorough discussion of this subject will, without doubt, bring forth many suggestions of value in the line of publicity.

The support of our schools and educational institutions is another matter for serious consideration. Without proper schools in which students can be properly prepared and thoroughly trained as practitioners and teachers the movement cannot go forward. Every practitioner and every person who has been benefited through naturopathy should pledge himself or herself to pay a certain sum annually for the support of our educational institutions as well as using their influence to fill such institutions with students.

Let us urge that when the A.N.A meets in annual convention from September 22nd to 25th, it constitute itself a deliberative body and that the delegates realize they are meeting for a purpose—that of furthering the movement for Natural Therapeutics.

> *The second consideration for the coming convention is to determine what qualifications a naturopath should possess and to make such qualifications necessary to admission to active membership into the association.*

The Clanging Doors

by Francesco Sanchelli, D.C.

Herald of Health and Naturopath, XXV(9), 426-428. (1920)

Dr. Sanchelli a broadminded man whose liberal views as expressed in the following paper read at the 24th Annual Convention of the A.N.A, have endeared him to all those who are working toward the allegiance of all factions in the interest of Medical Freedom. —Ed.

On page 46 of the August issue of "Physical Culture", Bernarr Macfadden presents a striking—a humiliating—indictment of every one of us assembled here to-day. On that page, in that issue, he says, in cold type: "The time has not yet arrived when the drugless practitioners can forget their differences and work together for a common cause."

If this statement is true, we might just as well call this convention off right now and pack up and go home. If we cannot forget our differences and work together for a common cause then this convention is a farce. If we cannot work together for a common cause, we are simply wasting time here and we are hypocrites when we come together in the name of goodfellowship.

It is hardly necessary for me to say that I do not exactly agree with Bernarr Macfadden when he says that the time has not yet arrived when drugless practitioners can co-operate with each other. The time HAS arrived; the time is NOW.

Mr. Macfadden has our best interests sincerely at heart. He has thrown himself, together with the wonderful propaganda power of his great magazine, whole-heartedly into the fight for universal recognition of the efficacy of drugless methods. He is our friend. He is our champion. He has made but one mistake; he has tried to please everybody; he has been too broad-minded for his own peace of mind. He has seen adherents of various drugless methods holding to their particular tenets with all the enthusiasm of a zealot willing to be burned at the stake for a principle. Small wonder then that he should despair of ever getting these zealots together on a compromise basis of co-operation.

Today I send this word to Bernarr Macfadden, the man who is working with heart and head and hand for the enfranchisement of the human body from noxious drugs—I send him this message today: Drugless practitioners CAN work together for the common good; they are GOING to work together, and are going to do it NOW!

Lack of co-operation among us has been inseparably connected with the bull-dog tenacity with which we have held to our particular and several convictions in the drugless field. Well, bull-dog tenacity is a great asset. Without it, we would never have won the grateful allegiance of millions of people to the drugless cause. When you stop to consider how we have had to fight every inch of the way to our present position of public recognition, you will agree with me that bull-dog tenacity is a very excellent attribute.

I hold it to be the inalienable right of any body of men whose general interests are more or less closely identified, such as drugless practitioners, to argue among themselves so long as their existence is not threatened from without and so long as their arguing does not at any time prejudice the interests of the general public. Right here, permit me to remind you of the paper I presented at the last convention of this association, in which I deprecated the practice of one kind of drugless practitioner belittling another kind, in advertising in the public newspapers. I held, and still hold, that this practice is prejudicial to the best interests of the general public. Our advertising job is to convince the public of the efficacy of drugless healing as a whole; they, as individuals can judge of which method they prefer, by the results they personally derive.

To return: When the existence of any body of men, such as drugless practitioners, is threatened from without, or when the public welfare is endangered, it is no time for this particular body of men to argue about the efficacy of their particular methods of achieving their results. Such a condition confronts us today. As a result, it is vital that we, at this time, fight in one single army, shoulder to shoulder, instead of in separate raiding parties—the term "raiding" being used in the sense of raiding the stronghold of the opponents of therapeutic freedom.

You all know, of course, that seven separate bills have been introduced in the Senate and House of Representatives at Washington, proposing to establish a Federal Department of Health. These bills were drawn by, and are sponsored by, interests that have but one overwhelming ambition in life—to put all drugless practitioners out of business. No one particular drugless method is involved; drugless healing as a whole is at stake. In this crisis, we must all stand together or we must be content to see the general public condemned to vaccination, to serums and anti-toxins, to drugs, pills and purgatives. The question is: shall humanity be thrust back into the torture chambers and the death cells of organized medicine after having had a glimpse of the light of redemption, or shall we fight this move to swing tight the clanging doors of medieval oppression against humanity's appeal for a chance to control their own bodies? To control their own bodies! That's what it means, gentlemen. Organized medicine is the Simon Legree of the 20th century; it seeks to control the living, breathing bodies of helpless humanity. Shall we fight against this infamous control? Then we must fight TOGETHER. And we must do it NOW!

I happen to be a chiropractor. I am not compelled to follow my profession as a means of livelihood. That is to say, I could enter some other profession. Before studying chiropractic at all, I was earning a very comfortable income. So I am not absolutely dependent upon chiropractic to assure immunity from the wolf which is reputed to prowl about indigent door-steps. Without doubt, every single one of you is in the same position as myself. You, too, could easily make a living in some profession other than the one you are now following.

Now, if I was convinced that chiropractic was quackery—that it did no good—I would quit practicing tomorrow. If chiropractic was quackery, and if I followed it as a profession, I would be a grafter. If I was a grafter I would get into some form of grafting more remunerative than mere quackery. But, gentlemen, I have seen the sick and afflicted healed; I have seen suffering relieved; I have seen racking pain disappear; I have seen the flush of health creeping back into pale cheeks; I have seen crooked limbs made straight—I have seen all these things as a result of chiropractic. And so I know that chiropractic is not quackery; I have seen actual evidence; I know we are giving actual, tangible, helpful service to those of my clientele. And down in Washington are those who, with all the cunning of the reactionaries of the Dark Ages, are intriguing with those in the high councils of our Nation to put us out of business because, forsooth, we are serving humanity! Down in Washington are those, who, preying on the credulities of the laymen, are insidiously seeking to deprive the public of the helpful services of chiropractors. Down in Washington, an effort is being made to swing tight the clanging doors.

I am only one man. My strength is not the strength of organized repression. Chiropractors, as a whole, are but one body of men. Their strength is not the strength of an age-old organization weighted with drugs, doubloons and deceit. But there are other bodies of men whose interests, at this time, are identical with those of chiropractors. There are other bodies of enlightened men who have been emancipated from the deadweight of drugs. These men are adherents of drugless methods other than chiropractic. I want to co-operate with these men to the end that this crime of medical oppression be not perpetrated on the American public. I believe I am safe in saying that all other chiropractors want to co-operate in this same end. I believe I am further safe in saying that adherents of drugless methods, other than chiropractic, want to co-operate with the chiropractors to the end that the clanging doors be not swung tight against the freedom of the public to choose their own method of protecting their own bodies.

I shall not presume to dictate just in what manner drugless practitioners should act to combat the threatened menace. Mr. Bernarr Macfadden has printed in "Physical Culture" a form of petition which merits serious consideration. But I do urge upon this convention that steps be taken here and now for concerted action of all the drugless practitioners to the end that the public shall remain free and that the clanging doors shall not be swung tight in their expectant faces.

Editorials: Diagnosis

Benedict Lust

———

History Of The Naturopathic Movement

Benedict Lust, N.D., M.D.

Advertisement, May 1921 issue of *Herald of Health and Naturopath,* XXVI(5).

EDITORIALS: "DIAGNOSIS"

by Benedict Lust

Herald of Health and Naturopath, XXVI(2), 61-62. (1921)

We are rather surprised at the way in which the average drug-less physician shuns the modern advances in diagnostic methods. One of the chief arraignments of drugless physicians by courts and legislatures is the accusation that they cannot or at least do not make a diagnosis of their cases. Of course, we are willing to admit that medicine has made a fetish of diagnosis and has almost entirely allowed this feature to overshadow treatment. A patient goes to the physician principally to be cured, but he has a greater amount of confidence in the doctor who makes a careful examination in order to determine his ailment.

Asking a patient a few perfunctory questions, listening to his heart, counting his pulse and respiration, looking at his tongue and possibly examining his urine for the presence of sugar and albumen, and then telling him his ailment is caused by "auto-intoxication", subluxation, eye strain, and telling practically every patient the same thing is either laziness, ignorance or fanaticism on the part of the doctor. Doctors are affected with mental "bugs" more than any other class. They are prone to chase fancies. Someone thinks he has an easy solution to the cause of disease, writes about it, talks about it and soon Mr. Average Doctor falls for it. It may be germs, it may be intestinal toxins, it may be orificial [sic] nerve impingements or vertebral nerve impingement, or mental aberration, or psychosis, or focal infection, or what-not. Whatever it is that the doctor adopts as his "theory" of cause leads to laziness in making examinations. One reason for this condition among drugless physicians is that they rarely charge a sufficient fee for examination to warrant their spending the required amount of time to make a thorough diagnosis. Another reason is that in some states the practitioners believe they are evading the letter of the medical practice acts by failing to examine or diagnose their cases. This, of course, is ridiculous. One may as well be hung for a sheep as a lamb. Recognition of the drugless work can only come through the thoroughness and efficiency of the practitioners.

My advice is: Do not avoid making a diagnosis for any fear of the law. The law will respect you more for your knowledge, thoroughness and efficiency than for your fear, ignorance or what they might term criminal neglect. Do not narrow yourself down to attributing disease to some petty secondary cause. Find out everything you possibly can about the patient's condition; for remember your examination is not only made for the purpose of determining causes, but also the extent of the effects—the state of function of the various organs or the structural changes that have taken place in the tissues. Meet the medical man on his own ground and prove the superiority of your work. Prove that you know all that he knows about disease and that you have better methods for assisting nature to cure it. Don't sneer at diagnosis and don't avoid it because it requires skill. Acquire the skill.

> *Don't sneer at diagnosis and don't avoid it because it requires skill. Acquire the skill.*

History Of The Naturopathic Movement

by Benedict Lust, N.D., M.D.

National President American Naturopathic Association

Herald of Health and Naturopath, XXVI(10), 479-480. (1921)

Naturopathy, or the Nature Cure movement was planted in America by the early disciples and graduates of Vincenz Priessnitz, the father of hydrotherapy, in 1845. American had already in 1850 28 water cure establishments founded on the teachings of the Priessnitz school. The Jackson Sanitarium, Danville, N.Y. and the Gifforth Sanitarium at Kokomo, Ind., as well as the Battle Creek institution, were originally "German water cure" resorts. In 1858 Dr. Trall, author of many books on hydrotherapy, vegetarian diets, etc., conducted a hydrotherapeutical college, chartered by the New York legislature, which had students from all the English-speaking countries of the world. Later on many of the founders of the movement, such as Fowler and Wells, Dr. Kahn, Dr. Baruch and Dr. Rheinhold, were well-known authors on hydrotherapy in New York City. Among the real Nature cure pioneers were Dr. Gustave Koch and several Socialists who came to this country in 1886 from Germany. In Chicago, at the same time, a certain Dr. Loewe became very famous with his Nature Cure Institution. Dr. Ludwig Staden and his wife of Brooklyn, Dr. Mina Kube of Philadelphia, Dr. Farkash and his wife were all conducting institutions with great success.

We ourselves came to New York City in 1892 and there were already in existence several Kneipp institutions, such as St. Francis Resort, conducted by the Sisters in Denville, N.J. in Rome City, Ind., Manitowoc, Wis. The Sacred Heart Sanitarium at Milwaukee, Wis., and Dr. Dodd's Sanitarium of St. Louis, Mo., were already well known all over the country at that time. From 1882 to 1892 there was a *Water Cure Journal* published in New York City which had a great circulation and advertisements from over forty hydrotherapeutical establishments.

Dr. Scheel and his wife, a homoeopathic doctor, were however opening on East 81st Street the first Naturopathic Institute called "Badekur," and it was Dr. Scheel who was the first to use the word "Naturopathy." In 1896 Dr. Scheel gave us the privilege to use this name in general for Naturo-Therapy, Hydro-Therapy, Nature-Cure, Physio-Therapy, etc.

We ourselves were commissioned by the late Father Kneipp in Germany in 1896 to go back to America to represent the Kneipp method, to start a Kneipp society, a Kneipp magazine, a Kneipp Institute and School, which opened on September 15, 1896, at 111 East 59th Street, on the site where the Institute for the Blind stands today. On October 1st of the same year we had already public meetings in Sassbacher's Hall on 78th Street and Second Avenue, which were crowded to the doors. The Kneipp method was very popular in those days. Dr. Jakob Riedmueller, Karl Klein, Eugene Stark, George Rauch, Ludwig Staden, P. Canitz, August Reinhold were our first associates in our work for the common cause of establishing and carrying on a drugless propaganda. Soon we found ourselves in difficulties with the New York County Medical Society, who employed a horde of spies, stool-pigeons, sleuths, spittle lickers and hell servants to embarrass the Nature doctors. At our society meeting we finally united ourselves for getting and protecting our constitutional rights. The number of drugless doctors was small, and as all of them were more or less Germans, who were not yet fully conversant with the English language, which naturally increased the existing difficulties. Dr. Scheel's wife then studied homeopathy and I myself was also forced, in order to maintain my work, to study medicine. The prosecution became so intense that we could not use the words cure, healing, therapy, therapist, physician, doctor or any other similar title. We were all in despair. Finally we decided to use the word "Naturopath" as being the only safe term by which we could designate ourselves as having to do with nature cure and disease. By this term we did not hold ourselves out as practitioners. In one year we had more than fifty arrests. The word "Naturopath" was the magic word that set us free. Although being a misnomer, it covered the subject. It has come to stay as a living protest against the autocracy, coercion, imposition, intolerance and persecution of the New York County Medical Society

Trust in particular, and the American Medical Association Trust in general. What the drugless doctors suffered in those days only those who were pinched can tell. The worst time of prosecution was from 1898-1910. Many a morning there were over a dozen drugless doctors lined up in the Court of the Special Sessions in the Criminal Court building, and each one found guilty and fined $250 for practicing medicine without a license. Chiropractic adjustments, baths, dietetic advice, exercises for the restoration or preservation of health was defined as medicine and a violation of the law. Personally I was arrested fourteen times and fined once $500 because a dirty woman sleuth of the Medical Trust with an unspeakable name took an electric light bath in my institution.

Our members and friends would do well by studying the history of the drugless movement for the last twenty-five years. We would like to call their attention to a reprint from an editorial in the *Herald of Health and Naturopath* entitled "Medical Tyranny in New York and the Persecution of Dr. Benedict Lust by the New York City Medical Trust." This will open the eyes of some of the younger men and women in regard to the sufferings and trials of the early practitioners. Same can be had at the headquarters of the American Naturopathic Association, 110 East 41st Street. Our practitioners who have come in from other States are enjoying the privilege of unmolested practice and this was bought with great sacrifices and personal expense. For eight years the brunt of the prosecutions was centered on me. To destroy our official magazine and to stop our publishing activities was their aim. Many Chiropaths pleaded guilty in those days rather than pay the lawyer's fee and go to a trial. But we are proud to say not one Naturopath ever pleaded guilty. Many in those years went to jail on the Island rather than pay money. The whole prosecution in those days was carried on on a commission basis, on the fines collected. In my own case, when I was sentenced, one of the three judges at the Special Sessions said: "There is no evidence that you practiced medicine or held yourself out as a physician, but we fine you just the same." But we did not lay low and came back on this combination of medical tyranny in New York City by publishing the real facts and exposing all their women sleuths, who for eleven years harassed and brought hundreds of drugless doctors to court on false evidence. One of these women would go to court, kiss the Bible and testify that she went into the defendant's office, took a bath, and while she took the bath asked the nurse whether baths are good for rheumatism, and as she said "Yes" she therefore charges the proprietor and the nurse of violating the medical law.

We have bailed out many drugless doctors and with our attorney procured often in the middle of the night bail to get a fellow practitioner —Naturopath or Chiropractic, it was all the same in those days—out of the Tombs. Finally, by a libel suit, we were arrested for exposing the dirty work of this notorious woman sleuth. We won out by proving to the court that this association, as a self-constituted authority, was exercising police power. Motion was made in open court that they should show the charter to the jury and prove their rights to exercise police power. They then offered a retraction, and after that the prosecution went to the Police Department, where it belongs, according to the law. That libel suit opened the door for Naturopaths and Chiropractors in New York. There has been little or no prosecution ever since. It is all over now but not forgotten. Some of our members served a year in jail; a woman drugless doctor committed suicide on the Island in despair, several died with broken hearts in the struggle and many happy homes were ruined. Millions of dollars worth of investments in institutions and other drugless enterprises were driven out of this city by the medical ring. Hundreds of drugless doctors closed their offices and went to other States. We trust there will be a time of retribution. The drugless healing art will go on, the names of these real pioneers will live for generations to come and this sinister power of the medical trust will be forgotten. The nature cure movement, Naturopathy with the fundamental basis of a healing art, *Naturology*, natural living, and with its sister the great physical culture movement, launched and championed by our big brother, Bernarr Macfadden, constitute a great revolutionary movement for rational medicine, a true prevention of disease, and combined with medical freedom, which we must and will get, it will usher in the new day of better health, more happiness and liberty for our bodies and souls. The nature cure and physical culture movements are the only popular movements for a broad education for the people on the prevention of disease. All other methods of healing, from allopathy down to the whole line of opportunity doctors to the fake gypsy Psychologist and Sex-Determinator, are nothing more or less but mercenary systems and enterprises impregnated with superstition and exploitation of the people. They constitute a menace to health and happiness and are unbecoming for the democratic and republican people of America.

We have every reason to celebrate this convention with joy, as we see the dawn of a new day. The rising sun of the nature cure movement will come into its full glory, will light in the darkest corners of official medical pseudo science, quackery, cruelty to man and animal. The fetters of compulsory blood polluting will break official medicine and make it a thing of the past. Our bodies and souls will come into their rights and future generations will exonerate the Naturopaths from the superstition of the dark age of our day.

Dr. Scheel and his wife, a homoeopathic doctor, were however opening on East 81st Street the first Naturopathic Institute called "Badekur," and it was Dr. Scheel who was the first to use the word "Naturopathy."

The word "Naturopath" was the magic word that set us free. Although being a misnomer, it covered the subject. It has come to stay as a living protest against the autocracy, coercion, imposition, intolerance and persecution of the New York County Medical Society Trust in particular, and the American Medical Association Trust in general.

The Menace Of The American Medical Association
Benedict Lust

An Association Of Free People Against Medical Tyranny
Diana Belais

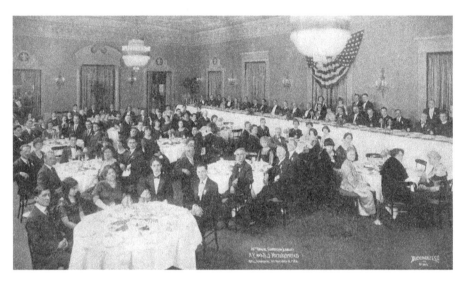

26th Annual Convention Banquet, N.Y. and N.J. Naturopaths, Hotel Commodore, N.Y., November 18, 1922.

The Menace Of The American Medical Association

by Benedict Lust

Herald of Health and Naturopath, XXVII(3), 111-113. (1922)

Order Is The First Law Of The Universe

About twenty-five years ago the American Medical Association felt the urge, obeyed the impulse and decided to set its house in order. At the time of this laudable enterprise, there were about one hundred and sixty-five medical schools in existence whose virtues and shortcomings were as numerous as are the characteristics of humanity. They ranged from the good schools to the obviously and admittedly bad schools.

The good schools were composed of both rich and poor students and drew their students from all strata of society. The faculties of these schools were composed of men who had a true appreciation of their profession. They were, invariably, men who were intensely sincere and honestly desired to alleviate human suffering to the limit of their ability. They taught from the sheer love of teaching and found happiness in their work. The students were, with the inevitable exceptions, imbued with like ideals. They studied—not how to become Golden Calf worshipers—but from the love of study. The Osler type of physician was their goal; the thorough, dependable, "all around" developed, human individual. Mercenary motives had no recognition in such worthy schools.

The indifferent schools, numbering about fifty, were old, conservative and wealthy. Their complacent graduates came from the better families—from the standpoint of wealth and Colonial blood. That such a combination lends itself to indifference needs no elucidation, abundantly abounds.

The bad schools, numbering about twelve, "graduated" students with little or none of the qualifications, educational or otherwise, essential for the successful practice of the Healing Art. Success in this instance does not necessarily mean the ability to profiteer. The existence of these schools gave rise to the phrase, "Diploma Mills," which is none too severe, all things considered.

Later on, the American Medical Association—by this is meant more particularly the Inner Circle of paid officers and presidents of some of the larger schools—decided upon a classification of all medical schools. This arbitrary classification, let it be distinctly understood, was not governed by principles of worth, integrity or ideals, but by the sordid conditions of wealth, buildings, endowments, libraries, paid professors and affiliations with State Universities, the latter being the entering wedge to State medicine!

This policy had the effect of suppressing sixty-five medical schools in the short time of twelve years, among them being a few of the avowedly bad schools, practically all of the poor good schools, and almost without exception all the sectarian schools. So it came to pass that there existed only the majority of the bad schools, the rich schools and many schools of inferior quality whose existence depended upon their connections as embryonic medical departments of State Universities.

EFFECT UPON THE COMMUNITY

Its effect upon the community has been far-reaching, the extent of which is hardly credible even after thorough investigation. To put it mildly, it is enlightening. Every effort, open, unfair or hidden, has been made, and is being made to discredit all Medical Schools not having a place in the A. M. A.'s select list. Irrespective of the worth of many schools, unless they be "acceptable" to the dictatorship of the Inner Circle, are unceasingly and unscrupulously made to appear unworthy in the estimation of the public. Propaganda, cleverly written, often ruthlessly discarding the truth, and paid for by public funds, are some of the means employed. Failing this, **special class legislation whenever possible is enacted.** Truly a clear cut example of abuse which so often is the offspring of misplaced power.

The majority of young physicians have been drawn from wealthy and well-to-do families. These upon graduation follow the line of least resistance and choose the easier way by locating in the larger cities. Many of them become so-called specialists. This may explain the phenomena of so many mentally-astigmatic practitioners, who see in every patient a huge pathological ambulatory stomach, or a diseased heart, or whatever single organ of the body represents their particular specialty, and amenable only to their special treatment.

The visits to specialists, so-called and genuine, are not always as necessary as the public are led to believe. It may also be said these visits are not as productive of beneficial results as an equal number, or fewer, visits to a rationally trained general physician. The physician who is not led astray by every new theory offered the profession—usually emanating from "specialists" —is likely to possess a broader and more rational conception of disease and cure than is the practitioner who presumes to trace the cause of any disease to one particular organ of the body.

Not only has the total number of physicians decreased, but with a rapidly developing population, there are very few willing general practitioners for the 95% of people who compromise the middle class and the poor. Last year ninety-three towns and rural communities in a certain New England State could not obtain the services of resident physicians. All of which is rather poor incentive and example in the efforts to build up the rural communities. It is almost a threat.

There is much wailing and gnashing of teeth over the alleged "officiousness" of the rural nurse. Many fervid prayers ascend to Heaven imploring a curtailment of the "pernicious influence" of the district nurse. One cannot eat pie and have it, nor can a policy which is rapidly decreasing the limited number of rural general practitioners justly say a word against the activities of the rural or district nurse.

Writers have contracted writers' cramp, reams of good white paper have been consumed, and orators have talked themselves hoarse in denouncing the alarming increase of osteopaths, chiropractors, naturopaths and other forms of healing, the combined following of which number close to forty million people! There is strong evidence of merit in such numbers.

ANOTHER FRANKENSTEIN?

If the American Medical Association, often called the Medical Octopus, continues its present policy, then in ten years hence, the good old family physician will be a rarity indeed. Should the plans of the American Medical Association be consummated, then the homeopaths, the eclectics, the osteopaths, the naturopaths and other "heretics" will be obliged either to emigrate, engage in some other profession, or become lackeys for the Medico-Politico Trust in this Land of the Free.

Tradition never intrinsically justifies a wrong. Injustice despite either its antiquity or acceptance is still injustice. The Inner Circle have been successful in having had granted to them huge appropriations which are used to destroy schools frowned on by the A.M.A.

The Russell-Sage Foundation, the Carnegie Foundation, and the Rockefeller Foundation are the chief bodies the American Medical Trusts have made alliance with. From these sources do they derive their greatest financial support in crippling schools not "approved and accepted" according to the autocratic and sordid standards of the Inner Circle.

As a people we are taxed, controlled, regulated, tagged, prohibited and exploited to the limit without the addition of such tactics. If only ten per cent. of the money spent in discrediting, crippling and destroy-ing medical schools not acceptable to the arbitrary barriers set up by the A.M.A. was spent in building up medical schools in need of fund, then in place of, say one hundred, **indifferent** schools, there would be almost double that number of **excellent** schools.

It is but a short step from State Medicine to State Religion; both are essentially alike in principle.

An Association Of Free People Against Medical Tyranny

by Diana Belais

Herald of Health and Naturopath, XXVII(3), 150. (1922)

Friends: This is the most important word I have ever said to you:

1. The large authority which the war has given the American Medical Association—through individual and Health Board adherent—has intensified its ambition many thousand fold.

2. This association of Allopathic doctors is taking immediate advantage of its increased power and opportunity by drastically urging compulsory vaccination throughout the United States, for adults, as well as for children, against small pox and even typhoid.

3. In one of the smaller cities the Health Board man threatened to call out State troops to enforce vaccination upon the entire population if they did not submit peaceably.

4. Try to understand what this means—this coalition of the medical and the military. When the Allopathic Health Officials feel they can secure, upon request, the action of the State's military arm, the situation is serious beyond words.

5. Nothing but positive public action will serve. We must move concertedly and immediately if we hope to retain our constitutional rights.

6. I invite all Anti-Vaccinationists, Anti-Vivisectionists, Homeopaths, Chiropaths, Osteopaths, Naturopaths of all branches, Christian Scientists, New Thoughtists, Theosophists, Medical Freedomists, and all brave and honest physicians of the Allopathic School (who secretly denounces the machinations and conduct of the political doctors), to send in their names to the Open Door and enroll as active participants in an Association of Free People against Medical Tyranny.

7.   No dues will be attached—but you will be asked to declared yourselves as resisting the grave menace of a medical association that is willing to commandeer military assistance in order to attain its autocratic ends.

Dear Co-workers, respond quickly to this appeal: Realize the danger of the situation: Unless we all act together and at once, our liberties will be wrested from us by this medical despotism.

Diana Belais, President
Editor of the Open Door

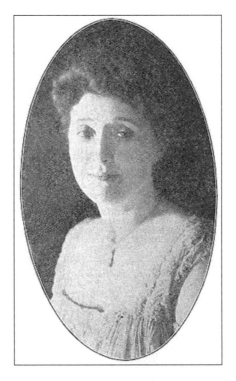

Diana Belais, President of the New York Anti-Vivivestion Society and President of the National League for Medical Freedom.

1923

Patients!—Take It straight Or Not At All
Benj. Israel, N.D., D.C.

———

Naturopaths, Forward!
Herbert M. Shelton, N.D.

———

Let Us Standardize The Practice Of Naturopathy
E. W. Cordingley, N.D., D.N.Sc.

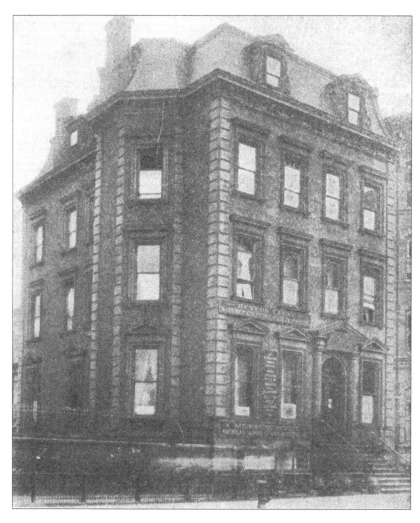

Benedict Lust operated this 55 room Naturopathic Institute, the American
School of Naturopathy, clinic and hospital in NYC, 1907-1915.

Patients!—Take It straight Or Not At All

by Benj. Israel, N. D., D. C.

Herald of Health and Naturopath, XXVIII(3), 109-112. (1923)

In the September issue of "*The Herald of Health,*" under the title, "Mixers No Longer, Put on Individuality," a sincere attempt was made to arouse the self-consciousness in the much-abused class of Mixers. It was shown that the Mixer, as a whole, has much merit to be proud of; that the time is right for them to put on individuality and organize. There were some facts in that article which were not pleasant to any sort of Straightism; neither did they please all variety of Mixers. Also, in this article, I shall make no attempt to defend all of the many varieties of Mixing and Mixers, especially the ones born and reared in the Hatcheries of the Fountain Head. My opinion about some of the Mixers is not much higher than that of Palmer. There are many among them who are conscientious in their Mixing; it is these I am defending from unwarranted attacks. Evidently Palmer cannot comprehend a Mixer with a conscience; all he can comprehend is the conscience of the Straight.

In his recent reply to the article I published, Palmer tries his best to show that Chiropractic and Naturopathy cannot mix, and should not mix, but if we take the health of the patient into consideration, I still cannot see why that could not be done. If, however, we take the value of money into consideration, I can easily see where Palmer is right when he says:

"To the 'Naturopathic physician' there are as many sources of his parentage as there are methods to be followed. Let me enumerate just a few: Hydro-therapy, electrotherapy, helio-therapy, stretching devices, zone therapy, etc. Chiropractic to him is just one of the many things or ideas to be used. Why single out and give it special prominence in this name of a conglomeration? Naturopathy includes everything; there is nothing more to be added. It's all in that name. Yet, you do tack on that one name. Why? Chiropractic today is getting the sick well. The public knows it. You know it. The public is being educated to the fact at a cost of hundreds of thousands of dollars every year. Chiropractors (who are) spending dollars to all of the rest of the mixtures' one single, sole penny. To ride in on that popularity of that Chiropractic name, that's all that's tacked on therefore. And to that highway robbery I object. Either be a Chiropractor, or a Naturopath. Be one or the other."

Did you get that? The public is being educated to Chiropractic at a cost of hundreds of thousands of dollars. And now, we Naturopaths come along and tack on Chiropractic to our name, and in that way some of the dollars that are supposed to have rolled to the Straight, roll into our pockets. Is it not terrible? And to that "highway robbery" Palmer objects. I should say so. We knew it all the time. But let us analyze this quoted paragraph a little closer. Palmer tells us that since Naturopathy already includes many methods, many ideas, why include Chiropractic? The question is a good one, and he answered it partly himself when he says: "Why? Chiropractic today is getting the sick well." Certainly. It has always been the policy of Naturopathy to include any Drugless science that gets some people well, and so long as Naturopathy will remain broad and tolerant, its future policy will be the same: Any Natural Healing Art that is worthy of such name will always be a part of Naturopathy. And that is the main reason why Naturopathy takes in the Chiropractic as an equal member in the Natural Therapeutical sciences, because it has proved its capability to get some people well. What crime is there when a Naturopathic physician takes a science that can do so much good for his patients and employs it in addition to his other Therapies? Such a man should be respected, not condemned, because in having good sciences to his armamentarium he has his patient's interest at heart.

Of course, we are extremely sorry that our inclusion of Chiropractic into Naturopathy does not please Palmer. He is interested in keeping Chiropractic Straight; we are interested in getting the patient well. And if Chiropractic aides us in getting our patients well, we'll employ Chiropractic, whether thousands of dollars were spent in advertising it or not.

However, there is one thing Palmer forgets when he talks about "advertising" and "tacking." He forgets what the Nature Cure profession has done to popularize Chiropractic; he forgets the aid it gave Chiropractic in its constant fight with the medical trust; he forgets the struggles of others, besides his own, for Chiropractic. Chiropractic to him is private property; no one has any right to it but he. No one may accept it or defend it without his personal permission. But we claim that one has a right to employ Chiropractic Straight or in conjunction with any other modality, providing one has studied it and has the patient's interest at heart.

When I stop to think over the foolish fight between the Mixers and Straights, I ask myself the question: "What is it all about anyway?" this whole issue seems to me to be so superficial, so unworthy, so uncalled for and so unnecessary as to create an utter disgust for the one or the ones who keep perpetuating it. Why is the welfare of the patient left out of all these? If the patient's interests were considered more, and the selfish interests of a healing science less, we would have more harmony in the profession. Service, as a motive, would do away with many of the troubles that are so common in our profession today. The addition or use of any two or three natural therapies for the welfare of the sick is looked upon by the Straight as a criminal procedure. Why? Because he had been taught that the one healing art he has learned is sufficient to remove the cause of disease, what crime does one commit in trying something else? And if it is a crime, against whom is it committed? In spite of the insistent claims the Straight Chiro makes, or may make, we all know that the thrust alone is not always sufficient to get all our patients well. If the Chiro has the patient's interest at heart above anything else, he will attempt to resort to the use of some other healing sciences, to the employment of some other natural forces to get his patient well. (But Palmer will immediately stigmatize him with his pet-name – Mixer.) And on the other hand, if the Chiro has the interest of Straightism at heart above that of the patient, he will never use any other therapeutic force, even though his patient is in torments without relief in sight. But his Straight conscience would remain clear.

Apparently the Straight's claim that the interest of the patient should stand above everything else is nothing more than subterfuge, for his greatest worry seems to be: how to preserve and pickle Straightism in its entire Palmer Purity. "Let the patient be damned, we must have him take Chiropractic straight or not at all." A genuine Straight, if there is such, may see a patient poisoning himself from severe putrefaction, that needs instant relief by an enema; or he may see one starving for lack of mineral elements in his food, yet he will not prescribe or give the relief needed for fear of mixing. It is to laugh to what absurd state of affairs the conscience of a healing science can reach under one leader's guidance. If he had his way he would discard to oblivion all other healing sciences except the Thrust.

However, that does not mean that we are of those who imagine that everything that originates in the Fountain Head carries with it a false and selfish motive. In criticizing the Mixers, the Straight Chiro tells many a truth. Many of the ideas that Palmer is broadcasting are undoubtedly sincere and well meant. Nevertheless, the few bits of truth, coming from the mouthpiece of Straightism, are too few and far between to serve him as an excuse for the many superficial, illogical, false and even slanderous statements, which he delights in making about many things relating to the Drugless profession. Under the false and misleading terms of Mixing and Mixer, created to suit his purposes, he heaps abuses on everything, or anybody who will not do his bidding. How long can the Drugless profession tolerate his fanatical impositions? And granted that he is sincere, should such a fanatic be allowed the right of destroying other people's beliefs and endeavors? Can the human race be safeguarded if we were to allow Fanaticism to be our only guide to real truth? No thinking person would depend on such guidance.

As an indication of his becoming an unreasonable fanatic proves his recent biased and uncalled for attack upon a great class or drugless physicians—the Mixers. We never had much love for Palmer before, but we respected him as a worthy opponent. Now, however, after our recovery from that most infamous and slanderous attack that: "An American woman is not safe in a Mixer's office," our respect for him is practically gone. We always knew that Palmer could use treacherous weapons against his opponents, but that one astonished us. We never imagined he would lower himself to such tactics. And as a result of his unforgivable blunder we are full of sympathy for him in a way. We still doubt whether he had his right senses when he wrote it, thought his fanaticism could easily account for it. Just think of it: according to Palmer, we are to think that all Mixers, in addition to their criminal offense of Mixing, are also trying to seduce American women. Is it not just terrible? What? However, we are somewhat cheered in finding that he did not include some other women besides American. It clearly indicates that the Mixer uses intelligence when picking his victims. Good for him. We surmise, accordingly, that in the office of a Straight only an American woman must be safe. Palmer says so. But what about the safety of other women besides American—are they safe in a Straight's office? We often wondered about it.

More seriously speaking, however, such slanderous remarks should never be passed without protests from the entire profession. Any practitioner who has a spark of manhood in him, including the Straight, should resent such false accusations against thousands of practitioners. Palmer should take back that statement and ask publicly for an excuse.

No other profession today except the medical seems to have so many spectacular charges and counter charges, challenges and fights, frauds and fakes as in the chiropractic profession. And why is it so? It is because the real motive behind their actions is not altogether the patient's welfare but his cash. I converse and read, listen and hear high discourses about This and That Healing principle, This and That Healing philosophy, This and That Healing Ideal, but what good is there in all that braganeering? It may ease some heavy burdened conscience, but it fools no one.

For our daily actions give us away completely. It is the dollar we are after and not the patient. It is true that the greatest principle and guide of a real physician if he desires to be honest is the welfare of his patient. His interest should come first above all others. If that were possible, we would soon cease quarreling; our energies would be turned to worth and value. Holding the patient's interests above others, the real virtues of a Healing Art would soon be discovered.

Of course, there are some of us, even today, who have principles and live up to them, but I only have in mind the average person, Straight or Mixer. Enough money in sight will create a metamorphosis: changing them from Straight to Mixer, and from Miser to Straight. Today, almost with every one, the acquisition of wealth is of primary importance. Were it not for the many economic reasons which guide our actions, there could not exist so many "two by four Healing Systems." In a social system where the urge for wealth would not be of cardinal value, many of the present-day artificially kept up divisions and fights in the healing profession could not exist. Our primary incentive would be justice and truth, not power and wealth.

As an example of how commercialism has created our present-day conglomeration in the Drugless profession, let us examine the many varieties of mechanical therapies, which exist as separate systems, for no other reason than their impossibility to come together because of selfish economic interests behind them. Chiropractic, Osteopathy, Neuropathy, Spondylotherpay, Naprapathy, Physicaltopathy, Mechanotherapy, Massage, etc. Each one of them proclaims to the world its self-sufficiency for the correction of all mechanical lesions; each one claims to do better service than the other; each one, also, claims that some other therapy had stolen part of its technique. On the top of it all we have many fanatics in each one of them who cannot see any value in any other therapy but their own. But who is right? Which therapy deserves to be saved? And which one deserves to be neglected and forgotten? Which of these theories, philosophies and principles are right and which are wrong? It is evident that under our present commercial circumstances such questions cannot be settled satisfactorily to all concerned, for that would lead us to investigate the truth in all these systems. We would attempt to find out just what part of a therapy is good and worthy of perpetuating and what part of it deserves to be forgotten. That is what we really need. The time is ripe for it. Take out the best of all mechanical systems, put them all together, analyze and systematize their technique, throw out similarities and establish an all-around system of mechanical correction.

But could such a revolutionary movement happen in an economic system that makes the acquisition of wealth the main motives of our efforts? No. Could we pick out the best of Chiropractic, of Osteopathy, of Neuropathy, of Spondylotherapy and from many of the others, and create a real Mechanical Science? Would the leaders of these professions allow their good but insufficient methods to be submerged into one great system for the good of the people? Of course they would not. Do they not ridicule such men like Lust, Lindlahr, Macfadden, Tilden and Riley for their attempts to include all Natural Healing sciences into one great Healing System? If it is the welfare of the sick that is of first consideration, then what real objection could there be for such a move as suggested above? Such a move, however, will be possible only when money will cease to be the main motive of people's actions, and the motive of service will suppliant it. And that is why I say to the Straight: You are no better than the Mixer when hearing the ringing of gold; you should know that a Chiropractic Mixer, after all, is flesh of your flesh, blood of your blood, reared in the same cradle, brought up on the same food. He also says: "Chiropractic above all forever." And instead of making Chiropractic straight and sterile, make it efficient and worth while of the welfare of the sick.

Naturopaths, Forward!

by Herbert M. Shelton, N.D.

Herald of Health and Naturopath, XXVIII(11), 635-637. (1923)

A question that perhaps every Naturopath has asked himself at one time or another is "Why has not Naturopathy spread as have the other drugless systems?"

Naturopathy is older than Osteopathy, older than Chiropractic or Naprapathy. Yet these, or at least the first mentioned two, are better known than is Naturopathy. Why is this? It is not because these systems and methods are superior to Naturopathy. For it is easily demonstrated that Naturopathy is superior to any or all of these.

It is my opinion that the failure of Naturopathy to spread as rapidly and as far as these systems is due to a number of causes, part of which are the fault of the profession itself. It is to these that I shall give my attention.

To begin with, there has been a lack of team work, a lack of cooperation and organized effort in our ranks. Naturopathy has been practiced under more names than any other system. At its birth it was christened the "Water Cure". Later it became known as "Hydropathy", then "Hygieo-therapy" and later "Nature Cure". It has been practiced under the names of Massage and Mechano-therapy. Some Naturopaths have called themselves Physiological Engineers. Others have held themselves out simply as Drugless Physicians. Some are Physcultopaths.

Today our schools are turning out Doctors of Natural Therapeutics, Doctors of Physiological Therapeutics, Doctors of Physio-therapy, Doctors of Sanipractic, Doctors of Naturopathy, etc., all without any regard for what effect such diversity of names is having or will have on the standing of the profession.

Some man among us decides the name is all wrong or wants to start something for himself and a new name is coined.

We have schools under these names, then we have Naturopathic Associations, Drugless Physicians' Societies, Sanipractic Associations,

Physio-therpy Societies and others. The same is true of our publications.

We do not now, we have not in the past, presented to the public and the medical profession a united front. We have not worked together. And all the time we have wrangled, not over methods and systems, not over principles and theories, but over names.

We need to settle on a name and all of our schools should adopt that name, all of our practitioners should use that name, all of our publications should use and push that name. What the name is does not matter so much. What really counts is unity and cooperation. Let us settle on a name, one of those now in use or a new one—it matters not —and then let us all put our shoulders to the wheel and push. Let our societies all go under the accepted name.

Let us come to a common agreement on a name, let our societies and organizations unite as one large nation-wide association under that name; let our schools grant degrees of no other except that agreed upon. Only in this way can we hope to make real headway against the opposition of medical men, Osteopaths and Chiropractors. Only in this way can we ever hope to put ourselves before the public in a true light.

In the ranks of Chiropractic there is strife and discord. There is open warfare between some of the rival schools. But they are all Chiropractic schools and all turn out Chiropractors. Their papers and journals all boost Chiropractic. Their organizations are all Chiropractic organizations.

They do not teach Chiropractic under some other name. Their graduates do not practice Chiropractic under some other name. They do not advertise and boost Chiropractic under some other name. Regardless of what school they are from and what association they belong to they are all Chiropractors and all talk Chiropractic. They may be mixer, but they talk Chiropractic.

As a result, everybody knows what Chiropractic is. It is known the world over. Osteopathy is much the same.

But our system, our methods, no one knows what they are. We have adopted too many names. Just like a crook who adopts a new name every time he changes places or residence, so have we adopted a new name every time we entered a new territory.

It is time for us to cease our childish quarrelings and foolish bickerings and get together and work together. Why not have a national meeting of our various associations for the purpose of:

1. Uniting them into one organization under a new name.
2. Electing national officers to head the united associations.
3. Working out a constructive national program for the future.
4. Adopting a common name, which name will be used by all our associations, publications, schools, colleges and practitioners.
5. Adopting a uniform standard for our schools and a common curriculum. This standard and curriculum should not prevent any school from adding to and raising the standard. It should be a standard that no school should fall short of and a curriculum that every school should include.

Two names that are at present in use seem to me to be better fitted to survive, and to me it seems that one or the other of these should be adopted. These are Naturopathy and Sanipractic. This, however, is only my personal view and may not meet with the approval of a majority of our profession.

Our conventions should serve some useful purpose. In the past we have met and patted each other on the back, fed each other on flattery and taffy and accomplished nothing. The salesman has been there with his machines and apparatus. He has gone into the assembly room and delivered a long sales talk which had no other purpose than to sell his articles of commerce. No one was enlightened. This was followed by a banquet and everyone went home.

Each man advertised his school or his pet method or his course and every effort was put forward to make money out of the convention. Let us convert our conventions into something more useful. Why not use them for the reading of papers on our practice and for the construction of our policies?

One other thing we have been guilty of in the past that has not helped us to go forward and to reach the public. We have given too much of our time and energy to helping the other schools to get before the public. Where is there a Naturopath by whatever name he goes that has not at some time or other boosted Chiropractic? We have praised it and advertised it. Where is there a Naturopathic journal by whatever name that has not published many articles favoring and boosting Chiropractic? Where is there a Naturopathic School or College, whatever its name, that has not, at some time in the past, or that does not now include Chiropractic in its curriculum?

Chiropractic owes more to the various schools and journals of Naturopathy for its rise to popularity than the Chiropractors are willing to admit.

What is true of Chiropractic is likewise true of Osteopathy, Naprapathy, Neuropathy, Mind Cure, Orificial therapy, Spondylotherapy and the new Abrams method. We have advertised these systems and methods from their very beginning. We helped them on their feet; we helped popularize their methods and practice. We aided them in many ways.

And what did we get for our pains? These fellows simply gave us a kick in that part of our anatomy best suited to the operation and left us out in the cold.

Do the Chiropractors or Osteopaths advertise Naturopathy or Sanipractic or Physio-therapy? They do not. And they oppose us every time an opportunity presents itself. They oppose us in their schools, in their societies, in their publications, in the legislative halls and elsewhere. Today the Osteopath and Chiropractor oppose us more than the medical men.

Why should they advertise us and our methods? They are busy putting themselves and their own methods before the public.

Why should we advertise them and their methods? We should not. Our attitude towards them should be one of tolerance and mutual forbearance. We stand for medical freedom and are not afraid of their competition. We should be willing to let them go along unmolested in their practice and let true merit decide who will survive. Beyond this we cannot afford to help them.

We need to give our attention to the spreading of Naturopathy or Sanipractic or Physio-therapy as you choose to call it. We should spend our time, money, energy, voice and printers' ink letting the public know who and what we are, what we stand for, what our principles and practices are and in what way we differ from other methods and systems.

Why shall we advertise Abrams and his miracle machine or Coue and his occult nonsense? We have enough to do if we attend to our own business and do not try to father every new method and system that springs up.

A few years since we were as enthusiastic in our endorsement and advocacy of the "Violet Ray" as we are now for Abrams' new wonder machine. Why do we give so much of our time and attention to fad chasing rather than to further Naturopathy? Many times have I heard the layman laugh at the Naturopath for his practice of jumping from one thing to another. We are accused of being as much given to this habit as the medical profession. When are we going to wake up and get up and put Naturopathy on the wheels of progress?

The time has come when we should get together and stick together. We need unity and team work in our ranks. Every member of our profession, every school and society, no matter by what name it is called, should put their shoulders to the wheel and push with all their might. Let us help ourselves for a while instead of trying to help these other schools of healing.

They are all able to stand alone. They do not need our aid. They do not appreciate our aid. We are under no obligations to them. We can well afford to work for ourselves now. We need to work for ourselves. When are we going to begin?

I move that we begin work for ourselves at once. Will someone second the motion? After the motion is seconded, will the Naturopaths, Physio-therapists, Sanipractors, Physicultopaths, Physiological-therapists, Natural therapists, etc., all vote for the motion? If so, we can go forward as we have never gone forward before. Let us hear from those of you who are ready for such a program as suggested in this article.

DEFINITION OF NATUROPATHY

Naturopathy is the Science and Art of using such natural, vital and purifying therapeutic agencies as will enable the human body to cleanse itself of abnormal conditions and set up such inherent healing processes as will restore and maintain the highest possible degree of health.

Let Us Standardize The Practice Of Naturopathy

by E. W. Cordingley, N.D., D.N.Sc.
Herald of Health and Naturopath, XXVIII(11), 684-687. (1923)

In my conversations with various Naturopaths, and especially in my visits to their offices, one fact that has consistently forced itself upon my attention is that the practice, or perhaps I should say the OFFICE practice, of Naturopaths as a whole is badly in need of "standardizing."

What I mean by that is that there should be a certain more or less definite routine among such practitioners that is in some respects identical in all parts of the country and with the graduates of all Naturopathic schools. Although I do not approve of the use of any single system exclusively (such as Chiropractic, Hydrotherapy, Dietetics, etc.) in the treatment of all classes of cases, as Dr. Collins says, from ingrown toenails to breech birth without the addition of other indicated methods, nevertheless there is one commendable thing about these single branch practitioners, and that is, the public in general thinks of each one of them as some definite thing.

However, when we go among Naturopaths, and would-be Naturopaths, we find a great diversity of methods being used in conjunction with a theory that is common to all of them. What I mean is that one Naturopath will put every patient, regardless of ailment, through a vapor bath cabinet, another gives a general manipulative treatment, still another regards advise to diet the main part of his work, and so on ad infinitum. The result is that if you ask any number of people who have visited Naturopathic offices what Naturopathy really is, some will say that it is a system of baths, others will say it is similar to Chiropractic, another will think it is something like Christian Science, while one who has had a larger experience with such practitioners will perhaps say that there is as much difference between Naturopaths as there is between cats, dogs, chickens and horses.

Of course, we know that no two patients should be treated exactly alike. The treatment given to a diabetic would not apply well to a paralytic, and we may have to deal differently with an 85-pound woman than we would with a 250-pound man, but, nevertheless, we can agree on some common points and have, in a measure, a certain positive regime that is at least in part applied to each and every patient. If every Naturopath everywhere can and will do that it will lead to quicker appreciation of the Naturopathic profession as a whole, and will give all who have tried Naturopathic treatments some common "talking-points" in explaining the system to their friends. And the sooner we get people to consider Naturopathy as a certain positive, definite science, the sooner we will get them talking about and discussing our merits, and just that much sooner will it become recognized as the greatest healing art the world has ever known. And before I go any further, just let me digress a moment to tell you just why I know Naturopathy is destined to endure. Without any arrogancy, I wish to state that I am regarded as a pioneer in Chiropractic, having entered that profession at a time when even many of the largest cities of many States knew nothing of Chiropractic. I have also graduated in osteopathy, in mechano-therapy, naprapathy, and nearly every other single branch system that I have ever heard about. And also, although I usually keep that fact a secret, I possess the M.D. degree. It is, perhaps, natural that I should recognize some merit in all these single branch systems, but I have also tried to pick out their flaws and limitations, and having done so to my own satisfaction, I have come unreservedly to indorse Naturopathy as the greatest healing art of all, because it takes from all whatever is good.

Now, let us get back to our subject. Most Naturopaths use some kind of manipulative treatments. We know that manipulation will promote the absorption of plastic exudates, and by accelerating the circulation and eliminative organs will help to rid the body of morbid matter that every true Naturopath believes exists in practically every disease state. Therefore, suppose every Naturopath in his office practice should adopt manipulation as the cornerstone on which his practice hinges. I wish our good friend Dr. Collins would put his "General Naturopathic Tonic Treatment" into booklet form and offer it at a nominal fee to every Naturopath, and then I wish every Naturopath would make it a point to get it. That treatment, which is manipulative, would form an excellent basis of that part of a Naturopathic treatment.

Then, in many cases, it will be desirable to use some method of "adjustment" of vertebrae, and the Naturopath can use his own judgment as to whether it will be naprapathic, chiropractic, or mechano-therapeutic.

Next, I would consider Spondylotherapy, or concussion, for the elicitation of reflexes according to the method of Abrams as an integral part of each Naturopathic treatment.

To the foregoing, let us add proper advice in regard to hygiene, and dietetics without becoming "food faddists," and we will have what I would consider a most excellent basic Naturopathic treatment that would be applicable to every case.

"But," some of you will say, "electricity in its various modalities has proved of value in my practice, and vapor baths have relieved many stubborn cases of rheumatism for me." All well and good. Electricity is of proven value in many cases. So is hydrotherapy and a variety of other methods. But let us use these other methods as adjuncts to our basic Naturopathic treatment. If you want to use sinusoidal or faradic electricity for paralysis, or hydrotherapy for rheumatism, use them but use your basic Naturopathic treatment as well, and let your patient know that this is always a part of a Naturopathic treatment. Let this basic treatment be given to every patient, because it will benefit every patient, and furthermore because it is one of the most convenient forms of treatment that a practitioner can give in an office practice. Then select your adjunct treatment to fit the particular case. I am sure that if you will do that, you will save your time and heighten the patient's estimate of you as well. Then the Naturopathic patient will know, or think he knows, just what a Naturopathic treatment is. If he goes to a dozen different Naturopaths he will get substantially the same treatment, and that will give them a better opinion of what we really stand for.

Another thing. A number of those who take pride in being members of the American Naturopathic Association seem reluctant in having the name "Naturopath" painted on their doors and windows. Many of them, if they are practicing in a locality where some single branch method is well known, call themselves simply by that name, and leave all mention of Naturopathy off of their signs and literature. I am not trying to get you all to discontinue the name you have been going under, but why not place the name "Naturopath" on your signs as well as "Chiropractor," "Mechano-Therapist" or whatever other name you may use? Then, if somebody asks you how it is that you practice differently from Chiropractor Brown around the corner, you can reply that you also practice Naturopathy and give the inquirer a circular describing Naturopathy. I maintain that if you possess a certificate of membership in the American Naturopathic Association you should have that certificate displayed in a prominent place on your office wall, and I further maintain that if you possess such a certificate, it is not only your privilege but your duty to have the name "Naturopath" appear prominently on your office signs. Ten years from now we are going to see "Naturopath" signs in every city of any importance in the United States, and the practitioner will be proud to be able to call himself a Naturopath, because it will mean that he is a member of the most progressive and the most successful healing system in the world. Why not take the initiative and let people know now that you are a Naturopath and do your share in telling people of what Naturopathy is really composed? There is a certain group of men, such as Dr. Lust, Dr. Collins, Dr. Lindlahr, Dr. Gemamato, Dr. Posner, Dr. Caruso, Dr. Pattrieux, Bernarr Macfadden, Dr. Cold, Dr. Reilly, and a few others, who have been fighting for a place in the sun for Naturopathy for years, many of them sacrificing a great deal for the struggle. Let us all show our appreciation by getting behind them and doing our part to the extent at least of letting our patients know that we are Naturopaths and that we are mighty proud of the fact that we are.

Now, before I conclude, just allow me to recapitulate what I would consider the basic part of the office practice of Naturopathy that I believe every Naturopath can adopt with benefit to himself and his patients.

Here it is:

1st.　The general Naturopathic tonic treatment (manipulative).

2nd.　Correction of action spinal (and also rib and pelvic) lesions.

3rd.　Concussion at nerve centers.

4th.　Common-sense advice on hygiene and diet.

It is true, as Dr. Lust has said, that light, water, air, food, earth power, rest and exercise are the principles of Naturopathy, and we all know and appreciate the value of these agencies in the cure of disease, but they must be classed under the heading of the advice that we give our patients. Therefore, what I am contending for is a standardization of the tangible something that we give our patients in the way of service in the office. To that extent, I am presenting my suggestion for a logical uniform regime as far as the office work of a practicing Naturopath is concerned. If my suggestions and efforts will result in a serious consideration of this aspect of the subject on the part of the readers of this magazine, I shall consider that my efforts have not been in vain.

References

Bilz, F. E. (1900). Allopathy. *The Kneipp Water Cure Monthly*, 1(7), 125.

Brandman, R. E. (1913). The medical trust busy again. The *Naturopath and Herald of Health*, XVIII(11), 723-725.

Cordingley, E. W. (1923). Let us standardize the practice of Naturopathy. *Herald of Health and the Naturopath*, XXVIII(11), 684-687.

Day JR, Hoyle EP, *International Homoeopathic Medical Directory, 1911-1912*, London Homoeopathic Publishing Company, London.

Erz, A.A. (1912). Friends of medical freedom and voters, attention! *The Naturopath and Herald of Health*, XVII(11), 707-709.

Fritz, W. (1916). The history of the healing art in the progress of drugless therapy. *Herald of Health and the Naturopath*, XXI(1), 26-29.

Greene, J. M. (1904). Why we oppose vivisection? The *Naturopath and Herald of Health*, V(6), 121-125.

Havard, W. F. (1917). Report of the 21st annual convention. *Herald of Health and the Naturopath*, XXII(6), 322-332.

Havard, W. F. (1918). What does the A.N.A mean to you? *Herald of Health and the Naturopath*, XXIII(4), 368-370.

Havard, W. F. (1918). Stenographic report of the 22nd annual convention. *Herald of Health and the Naturopath*, XXIII(9), 764-767.

Havard, W. F. (1919). Editorials; the event of the convention. *Herald of Health and the Naturopath*, XXIV(12), 583-584.

Israel, B. (1923). Patients! Take it straight or not at all. *Herald of Health and the Naturopath*, XXVIII(3), 109-112.

Juettner, O. (1906). A plea for physical therapy. *The Naturopath and Herald of Health*, VII(6), 225-230).

Los Angeles Times. (1908). Another medical persecution. *The Naturopath and Herald of Health*, IX(6), 190-191.

Lindlahr, H. (1910). The anti-vaccination crusade. *The Naturopath and Herald of Health*, XIV(2), 129-132.

Lust, B. (1900). A brief history of natural healing. *The Kneipp Water Cure Monthly*, 1(1), 2-5.

Lust, B. (1902). A happy new year. *The Naturopath and Herald of Health*, III(1), 13-14.

Lust, B. (1902). Editorial drift. *The Naturopath and Herald of Health*, III(1), 32-33.

Lust, B. (1903). The origin of the Naturopathic Society. *The Naturopath and Herald of Health*, IV(1 & 2), 36-37.

Lust, B. (1904). Father Kneipp and his methods, *The Naturopath and Herald of Health*, V(7), 145-149.

Lust, B. (1906). Opinions of physicians concerning medical science. *The Naturopath and Herald of Health,* VII(4), 160-161. Lust compiled a list of quotations from various medical doctors.

Lust, B. (1907). New York's medical confraternity causes arrest of Eugene Christian, noted dietitian charged with curing human ailments without drugs. *The Naturopath and Herald of Health,* VIII(4), 137-138.

Lust, B. (1908). Bernarr Macfadden. *The Naturopath and Herald of Health,* IX(3), 98.

Lust, B. (1909). A family chat concerning our growth. *The Naturopath and Herald of Health,* XIV(1), 1-4.

Lust, B. (1909). Our new naturopathic hospital. *The Naturopath and Herald of Health,* XIV(2) 87-89.

Lust, B. (1911). Medical persecution of the fasting cure, *The Naturopath and Herald of Health,* XVI(12), 776-778.

Lust, B. (1912). Naturopathic news. *The Naturopath and Herald of Health,* XVII(6), 389-393.

Lust, B. (1912). Benedict Lust's health resorts "Yungborn," Butler, N.J. and "Qui-si-sana," Tangerine. *The Naturopath and Herald of Health,* XVIII(7), 496-500.

Lust, B. (1916). An open letter by Dr. B. Lust to the drugless profession of the United States of America. *Herald of Health and the Naturopath,* XXI(7), no page number was assigned to this three page letter to the naturopathic profession.

Lust, B. (1917). Medical tyranny defies the constitution of the United States. *Herald of Health and the Naturopath,* XXII(4), 2256a-256c.

Lust, B. (1918). Editorial, our schools and colleges., *Herald of Health and the Naturopath,* XXIII(8), 709.

Lust, B. (1918). Editorial, Naturopathy and the epidemic. *Herald of Health and the Naturopath,* XXIII(12), 917-918.

Lust, B. (1920). Editorial, who will give the first million to promote Naturopathy? *Herald of Health and the Naturopath,* XXV(2), 61-62.

Lust, B. (1920). Editorial, facing the situation. *Herald of Health and the Naturopath,* XXV(6), 269-270.

Lust, B. (1920). Editorial, a new use for the injunction. *Herald of Health and the Naturopath,* XXV(7), 321-322.

Lust, B. (1920). Editorials, things for consideration at the convention. *Herald of Health and the Naturopath,* XXV(8), 373-374.

Lust, B. (1921). Editorials, diagnosis. *Herald of Health and the Naturopath,* XXVI(2), 61-62.

Lust, B. (1921). History of the naturopathic movement. *Herald of Health and the Naturopath,* XXVI(10), 479-480.

Lust, B. (1922). The menace of the American Medical Association. *Herald of Health and the Naturopath,* XXV(3), 111-113.

Macfadden, B. (1919). Shall we have medical freedom? *Herald of Health and the Naturopath,* XXIV(7), 336-337.

Mann, H. (1905). Our medical laws. *The Naturopath and Herald of Health,* VI(6), 158-160.

Miller, T. (2013). Obesity is officially a disease, American Medical Association rules. *New York Daily News,* June 19, 2013. Accessed: www. nydailynews.com/life-style/health/obesity-fficially-disease-american-medical-association-rules-article-1.1376796.

New York State Society of Naturopaths. (1914). Naturopathic legislation series, part one, brief I, II, and III. The *Naturopath and Herald of Health,* XIX(3), 143-150.

Purinton, E. E. (1915). Efficiency in drugless healing, a year of triumph. *The Naturopath and Herald of Health,* XVIII(7), 1-7.

Robinson, J.T. (1911). Something far-reaching. *The Naturopath and Herald of Health,* XVI(2), 106-107.

S. A. B. (1905). The medical "fakir". *The Naturopath and Herald of Health,* VI(3), 74-75.

Sanchelli, F.(1920). The clanging doors. *Herald of Health and Naturopath,* XXV(9), 426-428.

Shelton, H. (1923). Naturopaths, forward! *Herald of Health and the Naturopath,* XXVIII(11), 635-637.

The Ophtalmologist. (1905). Who are the quacks? *The Naturopath and Herald of Health,* VI(4), 61-65.

White, C. I. (1908). The defense fund. *The Naturopath and Herald of Health,* IX(2), 66.

INDEX

A

Ablutions, 89
Abrams method, 353
Acute disease, 122, 164, 310
Aerotherapy, 69
Air, air cure, 53, 88, 153, 175, 207, 219, 225, 281
Allopaths, allopathy, 55, 135, 190, 231, 261, 292, 297, 299, 331, 339
American Army, 213, 261
American Drugless University, 305
American Medical Association, (A.M.A.), 97, 136, 137, 169, 172, 196, 197, 214, 274, 303, 306, 335, 336, 337, 339
American Medical Trust, 300, 338
American Naturopathic Association, (A.N.A.), 253, 255, 257, 265, 273, 274, 277, 305, 317, 329, 358, 359
American School of Naturopathy, 148
Amerikanische Kneipp-Blätter, 65
Anatomy, 172
Anesthesia, 79, 82, 83, 247
Anti-toxins, 102, 310, 321
Anti-vaccination, 161, 339
Anti-vivisectionist, 79-85, 339
Arena, (editor, B. O. Flower), 170
Aristophage, 69
Arrested, arrest warrant, 129, 138, 139, 141, 185, 193, 301, 314, 329, 330
Art, 253, 303, 312, 313, 330
Aryans, 250
Auto-intoxication, 123,325

B

Bacilli, 55

Baconian philosophy, 248
Badekur, 69, 328
Bandage, 47
Baths, 43, 148, 191, 281, 302, 329
    Air, 52, 153, 205, 219, 228, 281
    Full, 90
    Half, 89, 90, 91
    Light, 52, 219, 228, 281
    Steam, 91, 250
    Sun, 52, 205, 219, 228
Battle Creek Institute, 327
Bowels, 48
Blood, 50, 51, 90, 163, 204, 207, 208, 264, 310
Blood-letting, 150, 175
Boils, 165
Board of Examiners, 135, 155, 297
Board of Health, 111, 255, 268
Breathing, 135, 148, 153, 195, 205, 207, 228

C

Cold water, 46, 51, 91
Calomel, 247
Capsicum, 250
Carnegie Corporation, 309
Carnegie Foundation, 242, 338
Castor oil, 247
Catarrh, 165
Chamber tea, 175
Chinese, 250, 251
Chiropractic schools, 172
Chiropractor, chiropractor, 157, 238, 247, 299, 304, 311, 312, 314, 315, 321, 322, 329, 330, 337, 339, 343, 344-346, 348-349, 350, 353, 356
Chiropractic Straight, 344-348
Christian Science, 59-60, 122,190, 236, 237, 238, 240, 241, 247, 298, 299, 339, 356
Chronic disease, 123, 164, 165

NAME INDEX

About the Editor, NUNM, NUNM Press

Sᴜssᴀɴɴᴀ Cᴢᴇʀᴀɴᴋᴏ, ND, BBE, is a 1994 graduate of CCNM (Toronto). She is a licensed ND in Oregon. In the last twenty-two years, she has developed an extensive armamentarium of traditional naturopathic therapies for her patients. Especially interested in balneotherapy, botanical medicine, breathing and nutrition, she is a frequent international presenter and workshop leader. She is a monthly Contributing Editor (Nature Cure—Past Pearls) for NDNR and a Contributing Writer for the Foundations of Naturopathic Medicine Project. Dr. Czeranko founded *The Breathing Academy* and along with Dr. Karis Tressel *The Nature-Cure Academy*, both of which provide training and practicums for Naturopathic doctors, the former in the scientific model of Buteyko breathing therapy, and the latter in traditional Naturopathic modalities. Dr. Czeranko also founded *Manitou Waters Clinic, Spa and Health Education Centre* in Saskatchewan, Canada, on the shores of a pristine, highly mineralized northern lake.

NUNM (National University of Natural Medicine, Portland, Oregon) was founded in 1956 as National College of Naturopathic Medicine (NCNM). It transitioned to university status in June 2016. NUNM is home to the longest serving, accredited clinical doctorate naturopathic program in North America and to numerous accredited graduate research programs and undergraduate programs. NUNM's program mix also includes one of the country's most unique clinical doctorates in Classical Chinese Medicine.

NUNM Press publishes distinctive titles that enrich the history, clinical practice, and contemporary significance of natural medicine traditions. The rare book collection on natural medicine at NUNM is the largest and most complete of its kind in North America and is the primary source for this landmark series— *In Their Own Words*—which brings to life and timely relevance the very best of early naturopathic literature.

The Hevert Collection: *In Their Own Words*
A Twelve-book Series

Origins of Naturopathic Medicine

Philosophy of Naturopathic Medicine

Dietetics of Naturopathic Medicine

Principles of Naturopathic Medicine

Practice of Naturopathic Medicine

Vaccination and Naturopathic Medicine

Physical Culture in Naturopathic Medicine

Herbs in Naturopathic Medicine

Mental Culture in Naturopathic Medicine

Water Cure in Naturopathic Medicine

Clinical Pearls of Naturopathic Medicine, Vol. I

Clinical Pearls of Naturopathic Medicine, Vol. II

From the NUNM Rare Book Collection On Natural Medicine.
Published By NUNM Press, Portland, Oregon.